The Charm of Castles

A Seasonal Exploration

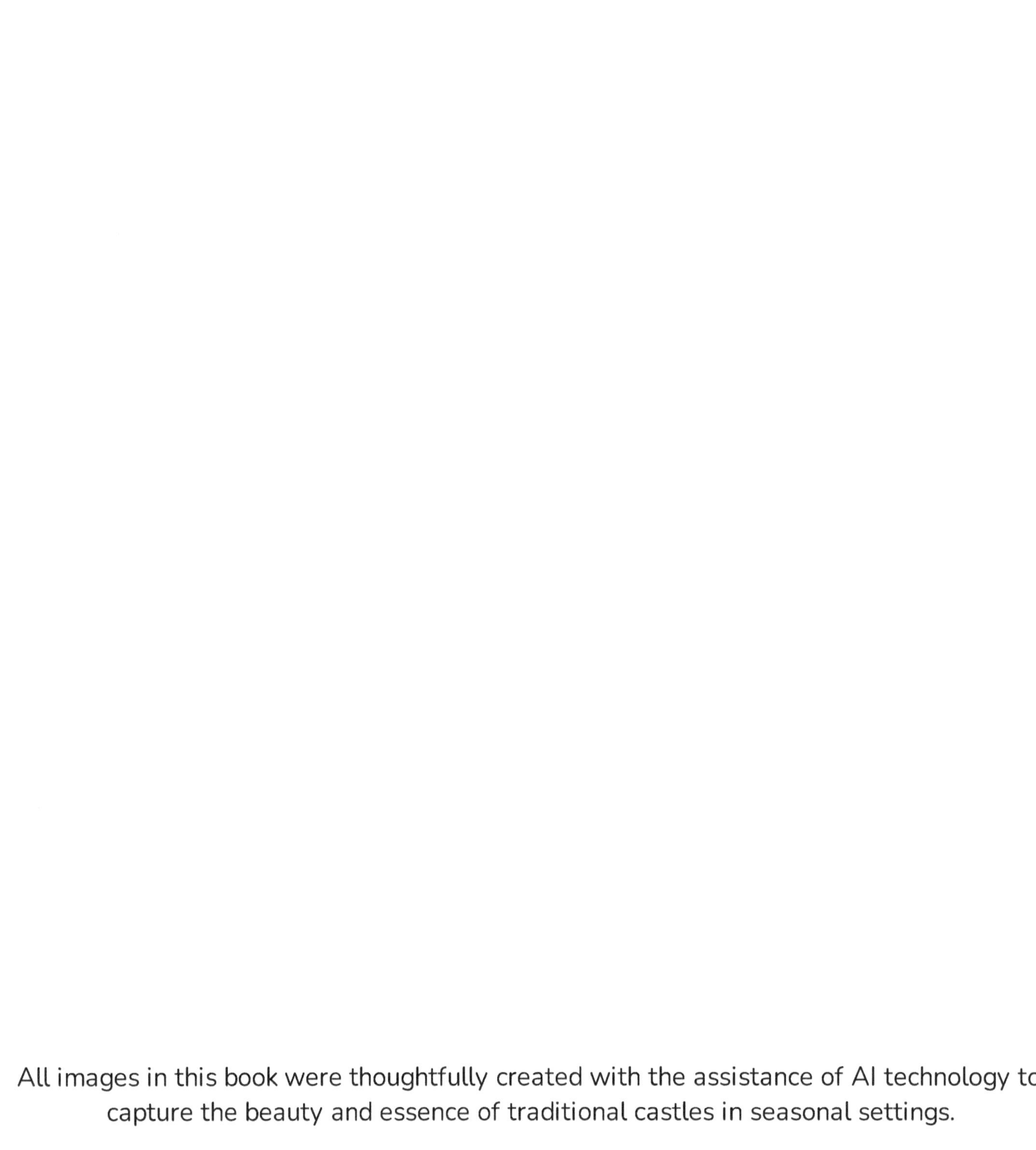

All images in this book were thoughtfully created with the assistance of AI technology to capture the beauty and essence of traditional castles in seasonal settings.

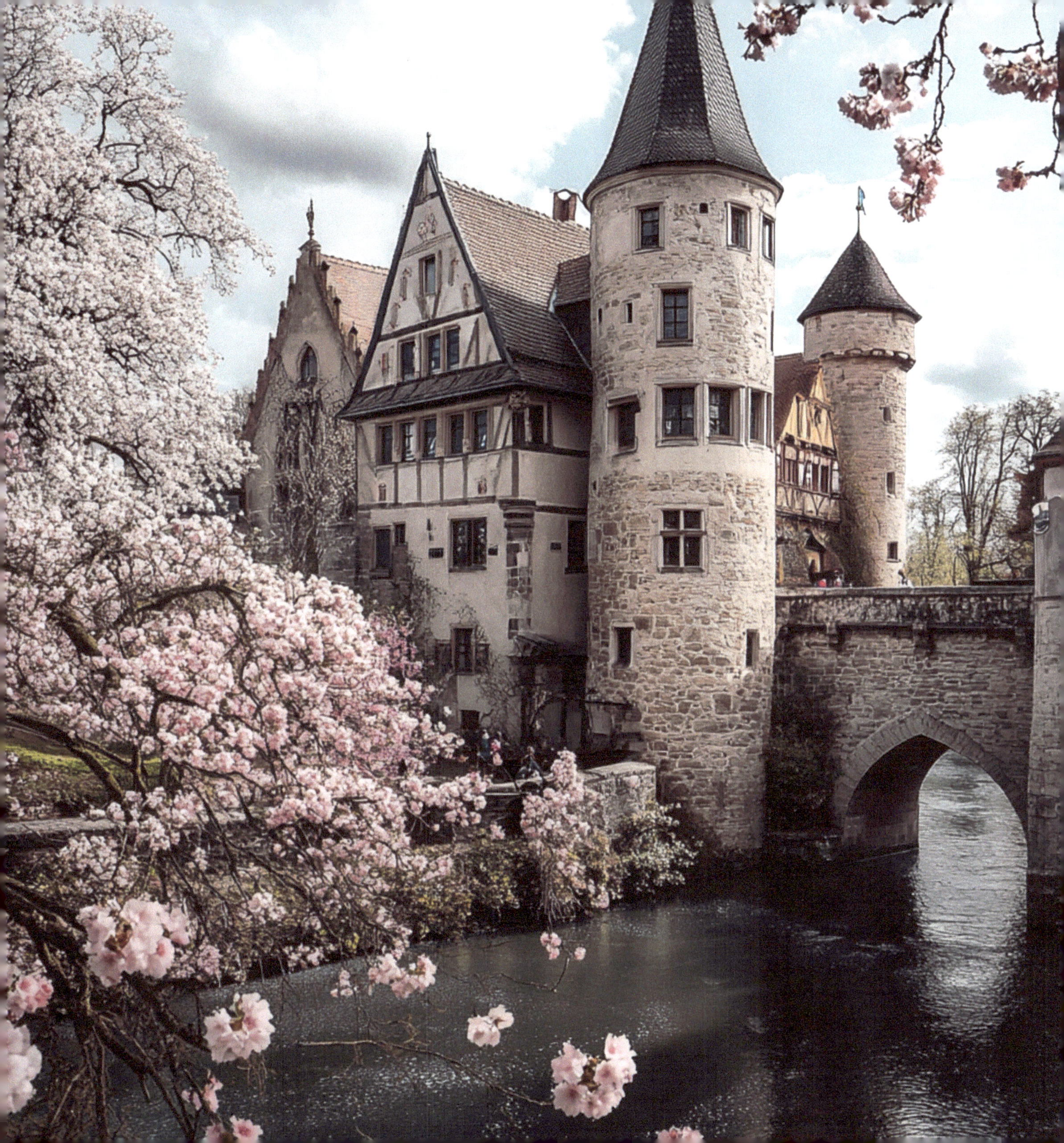

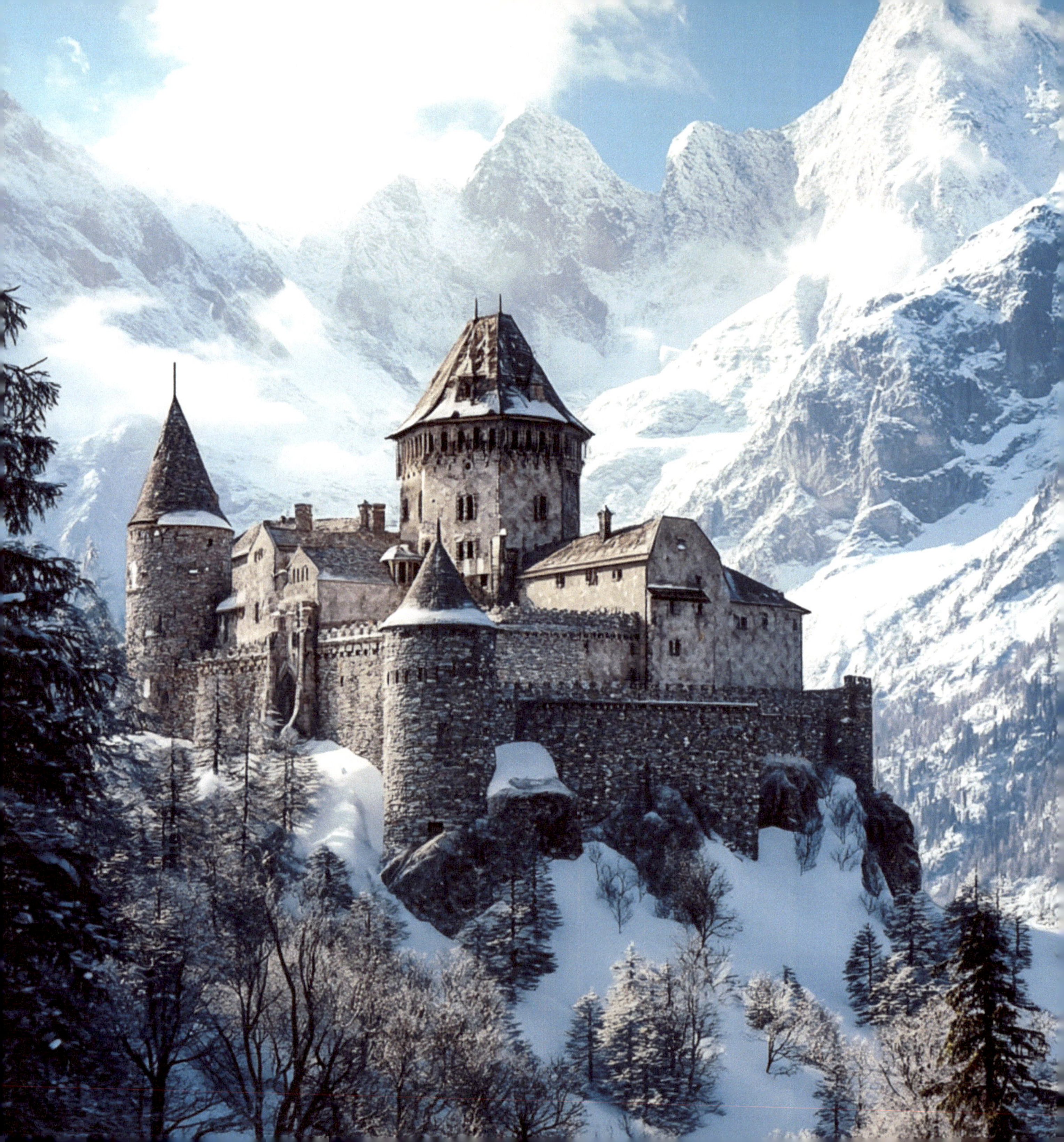

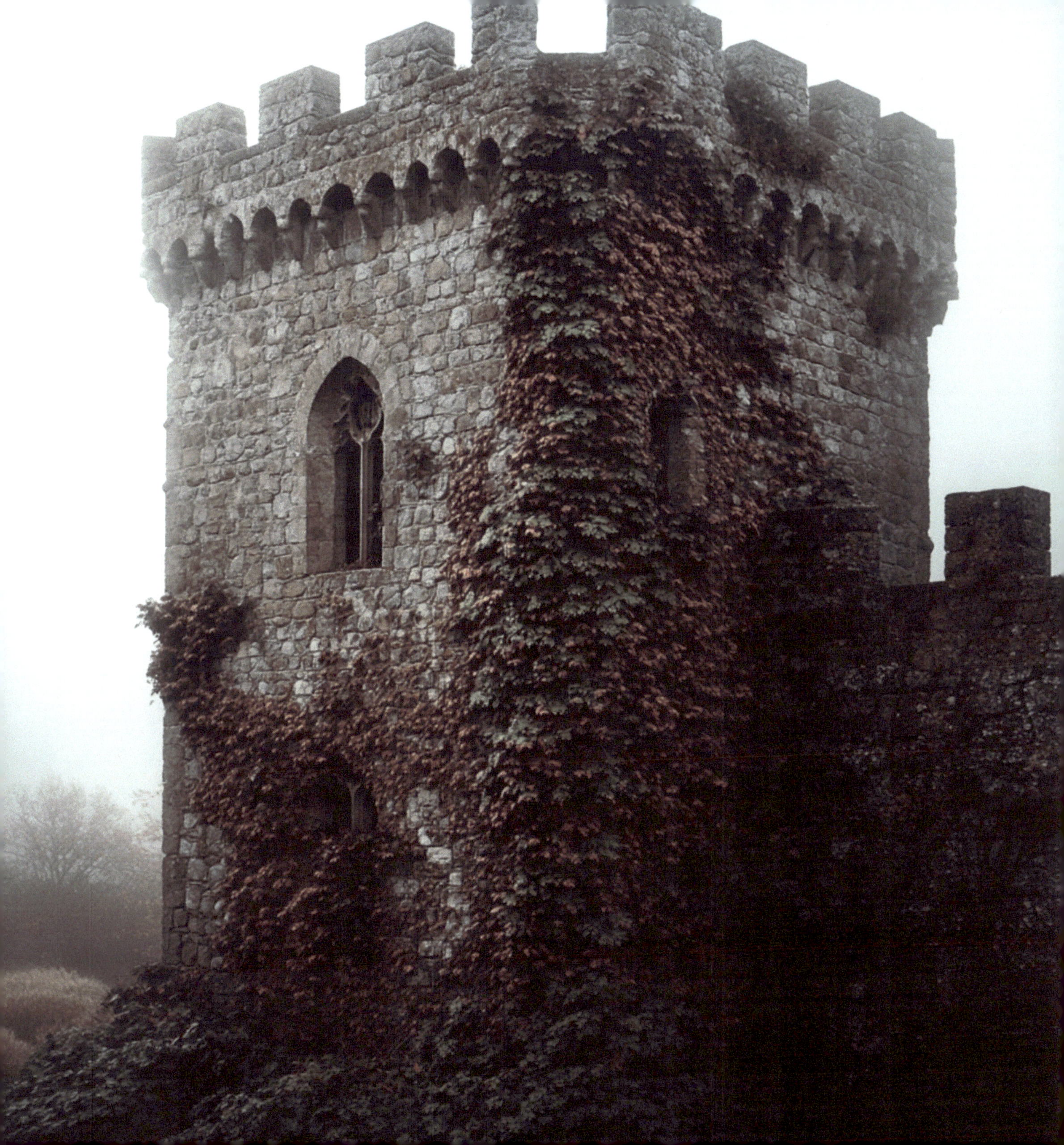

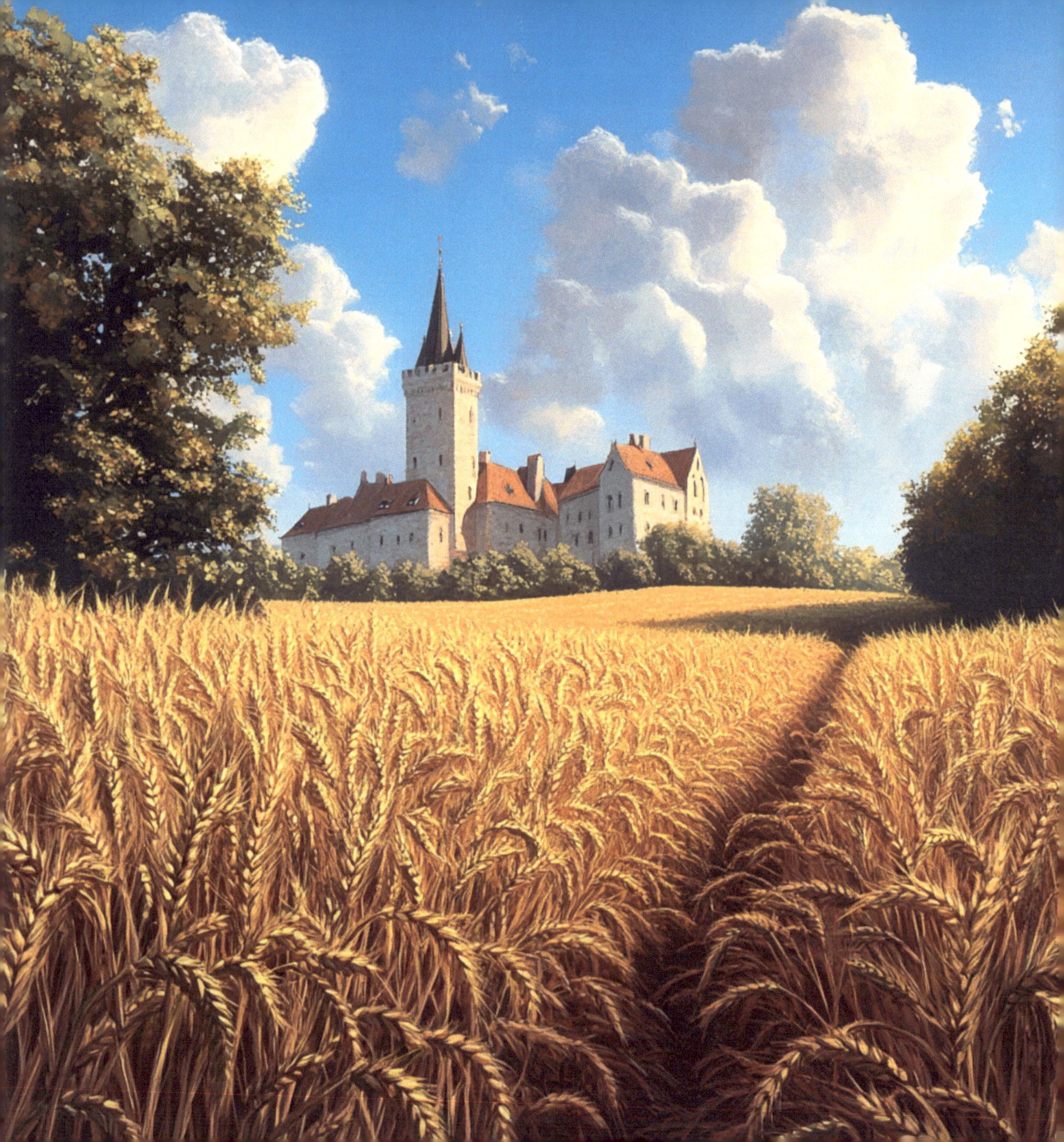

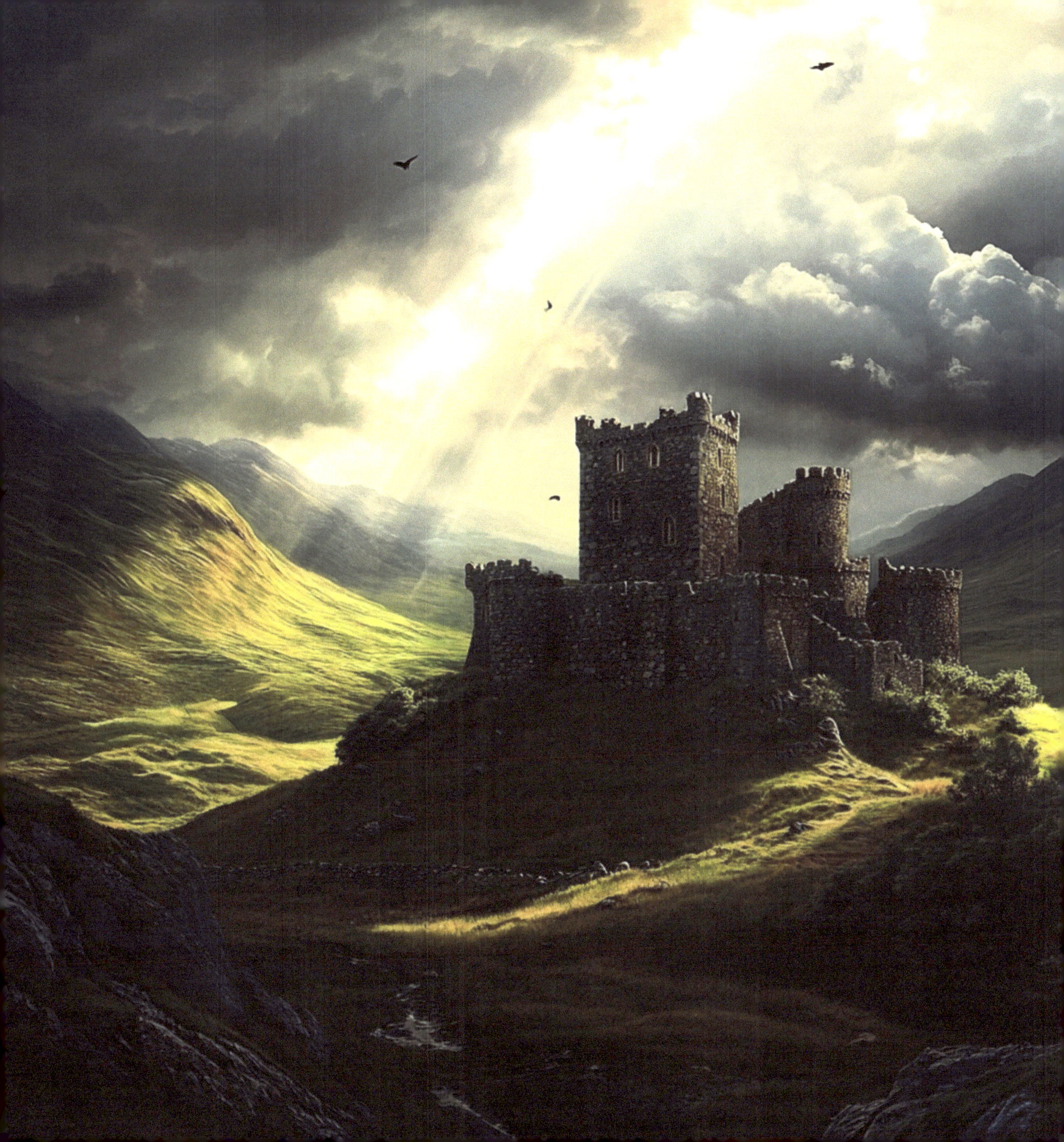

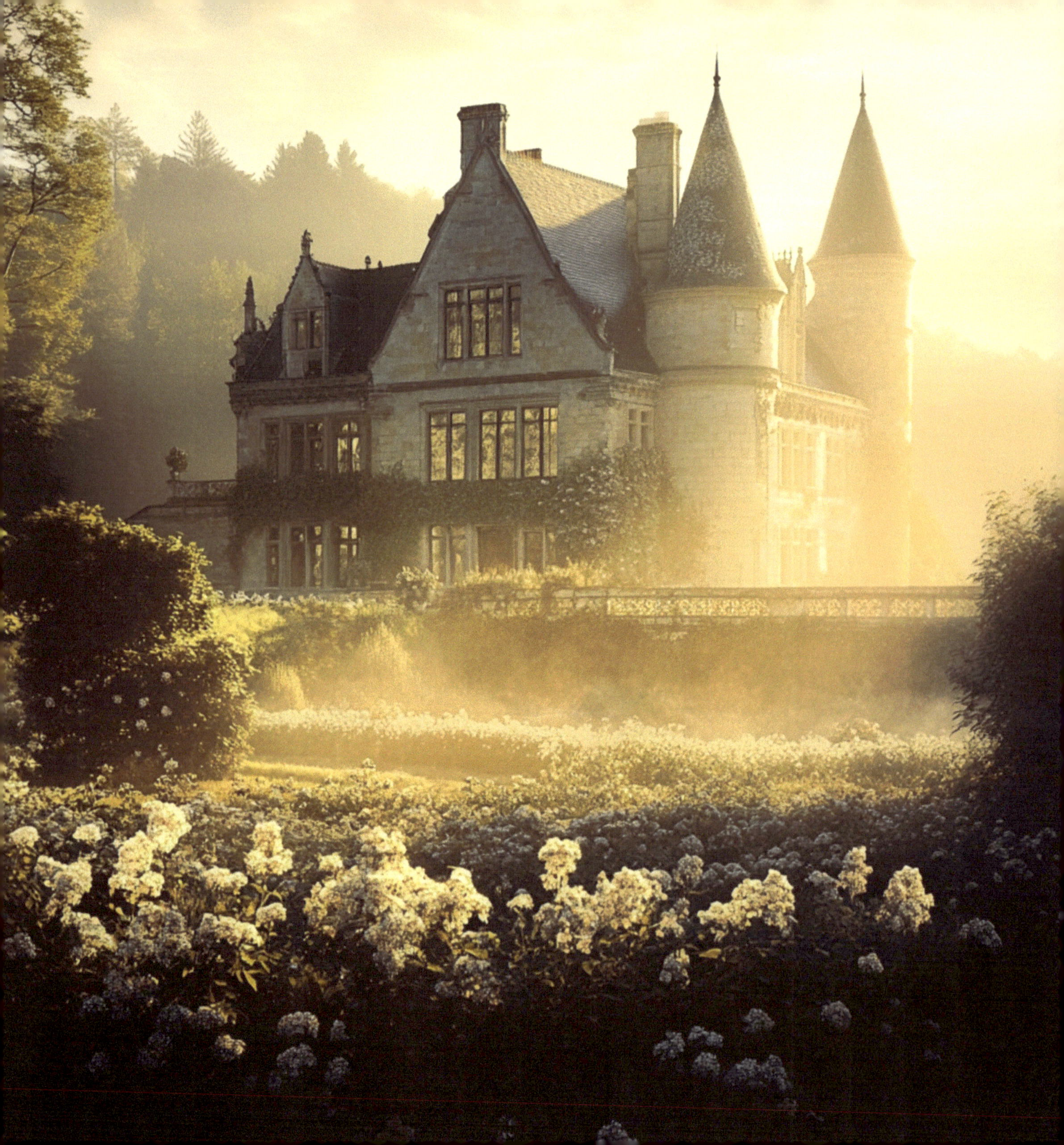

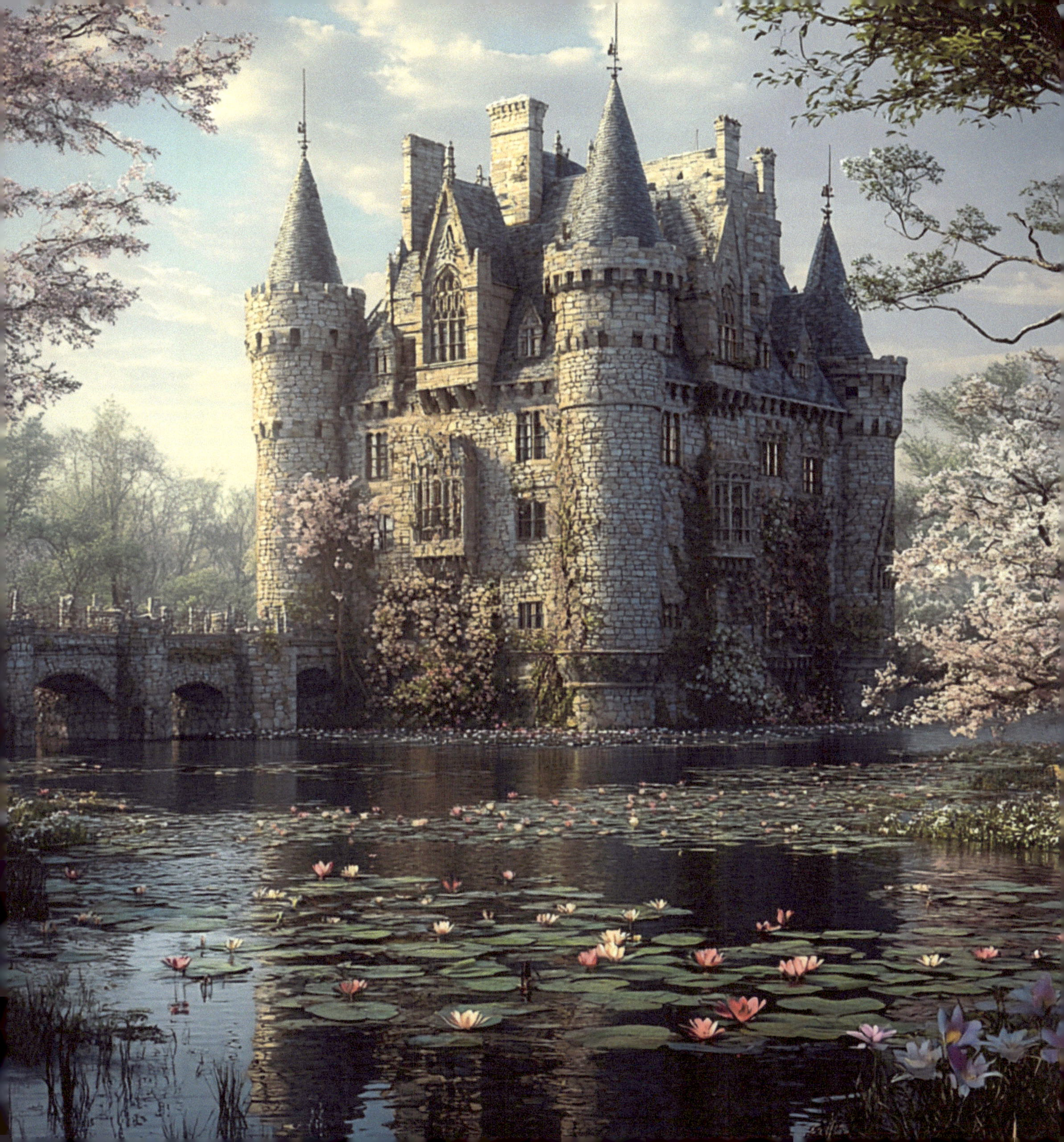

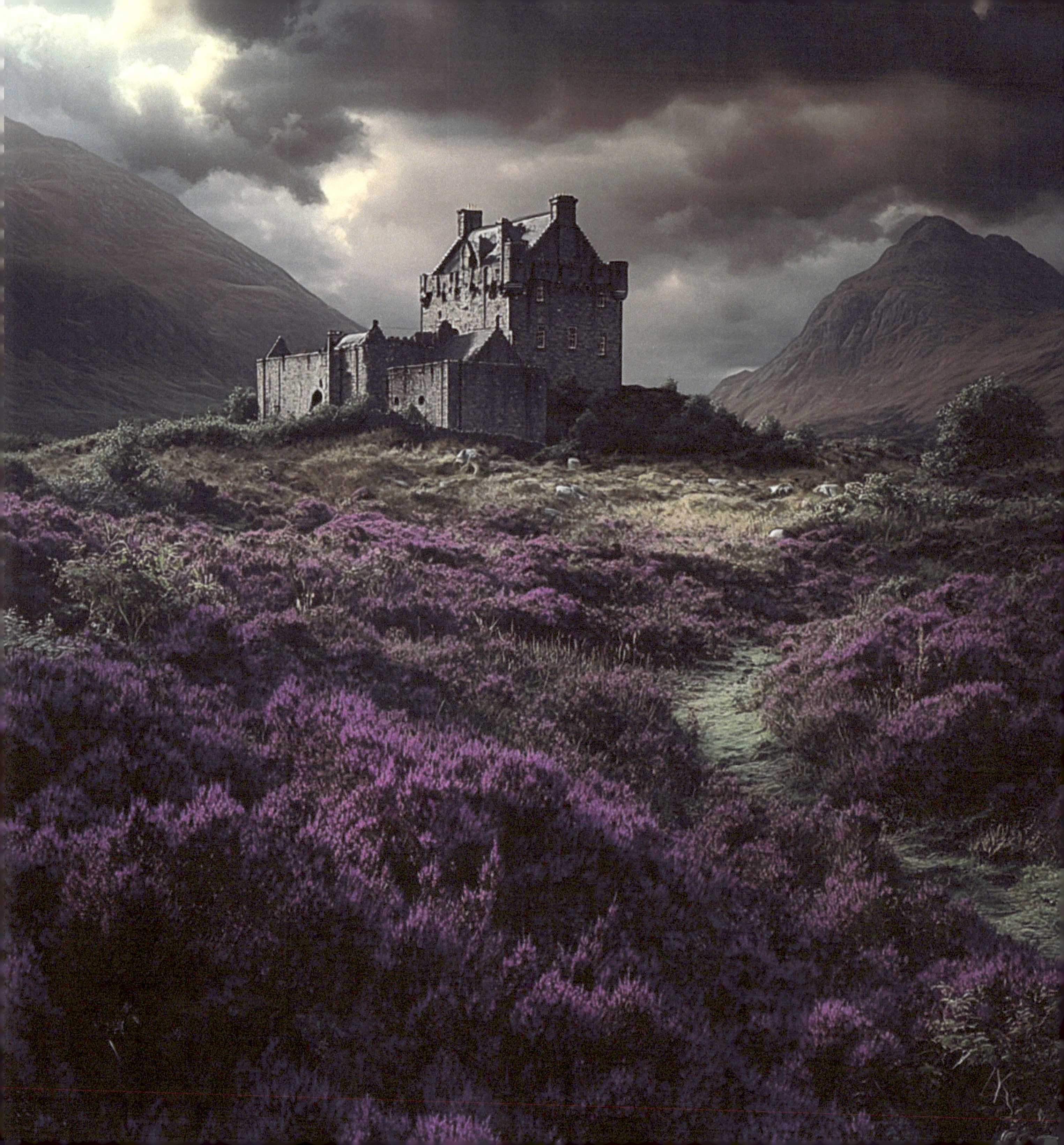

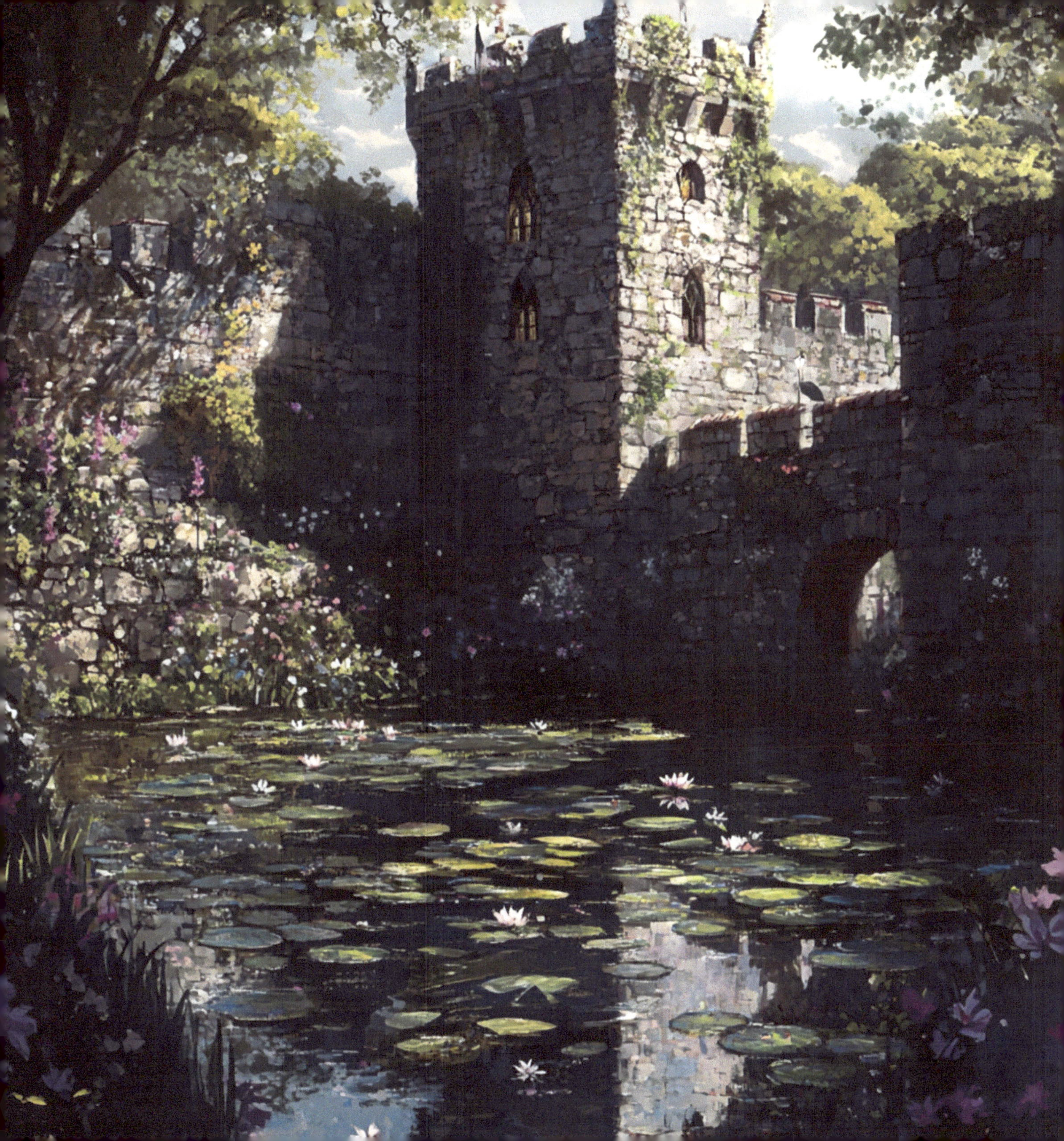

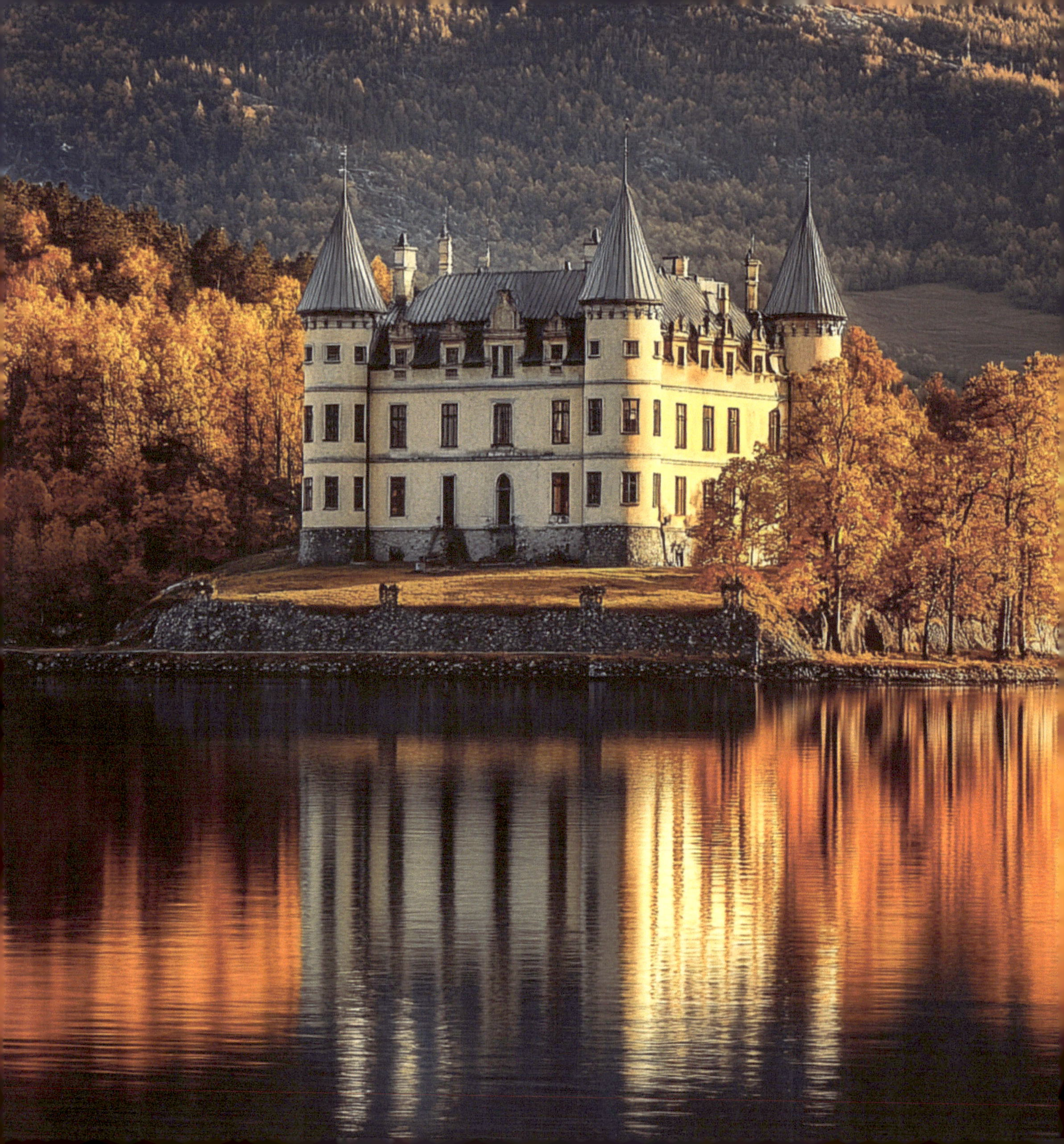

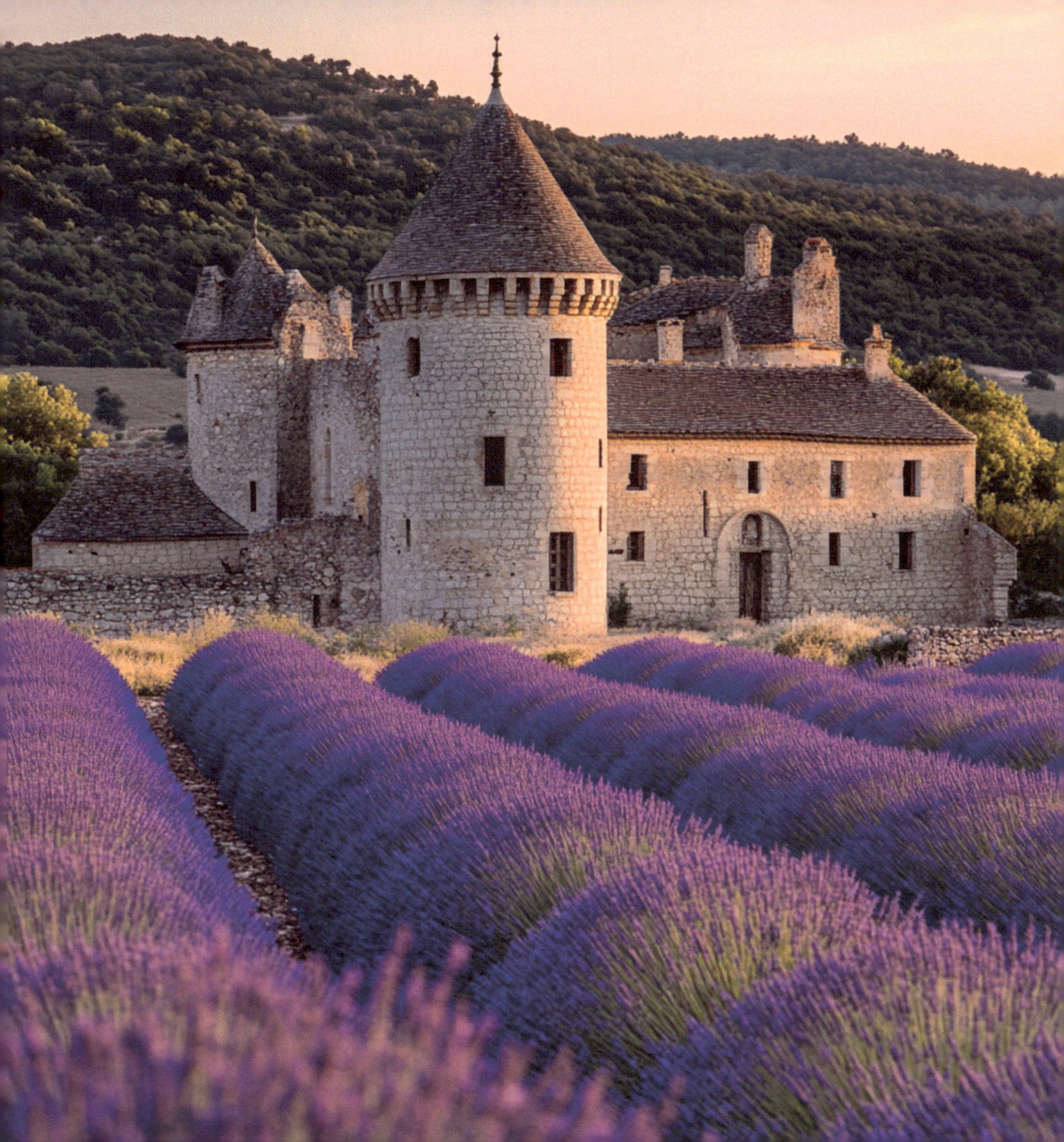

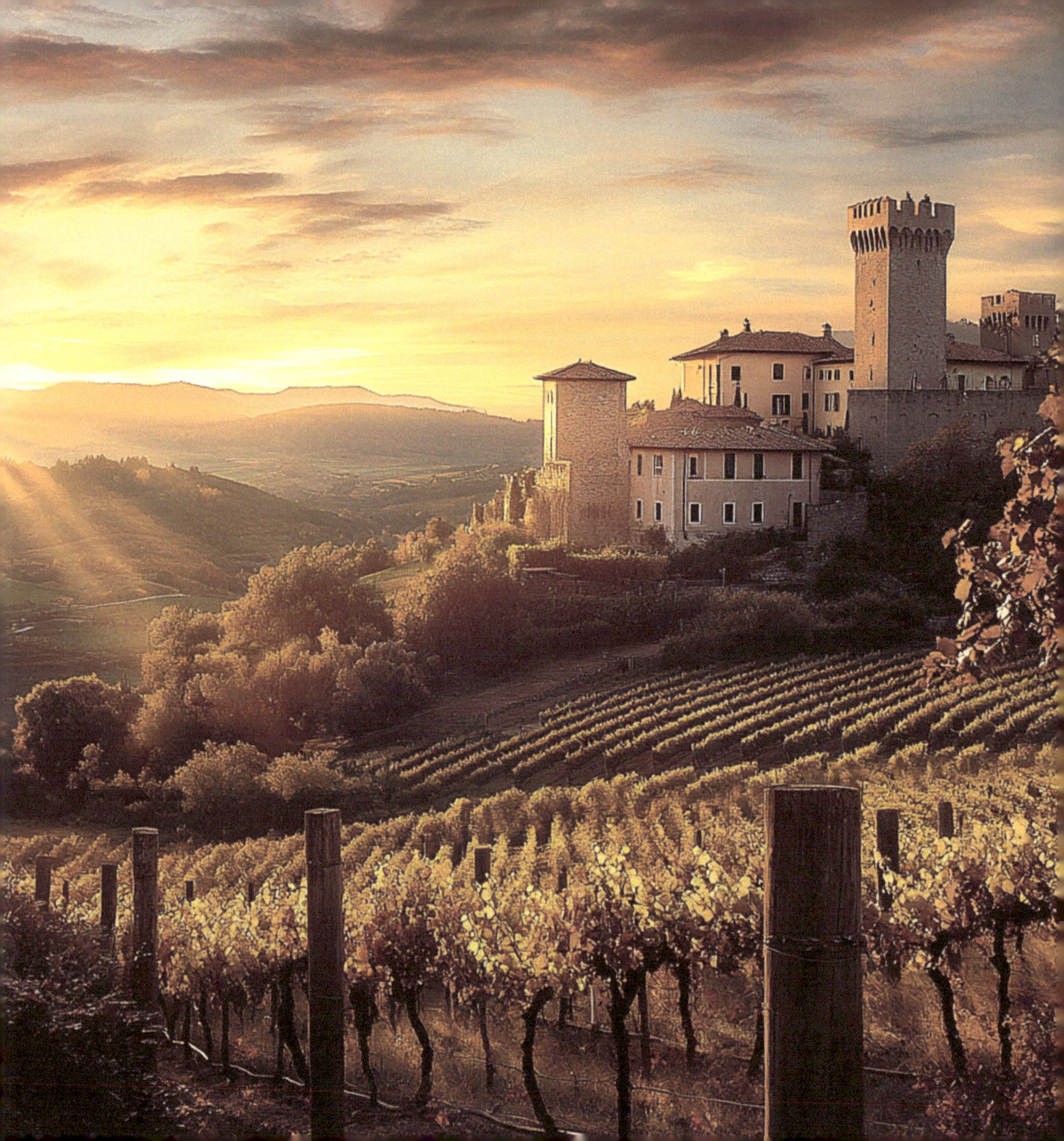

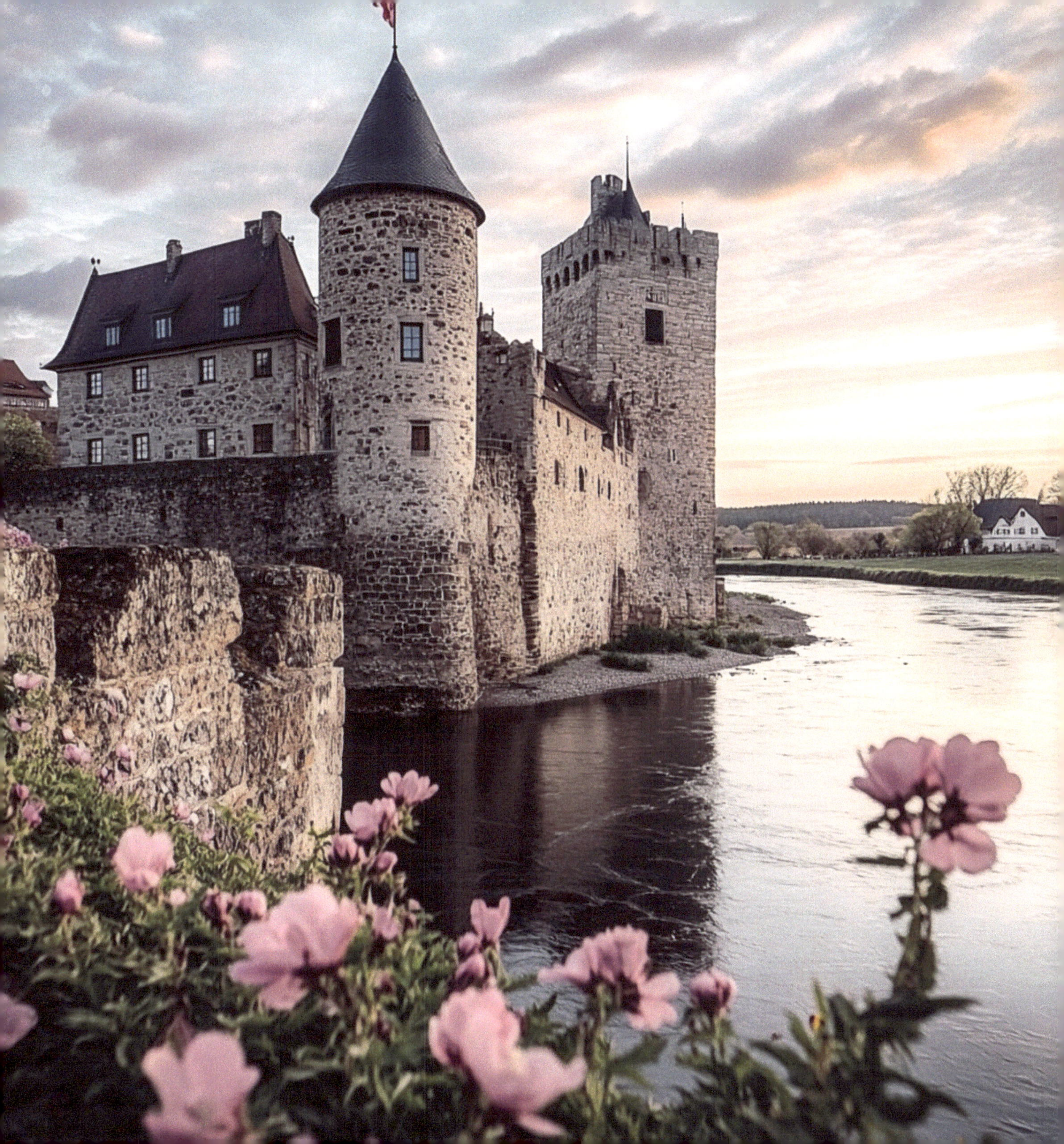

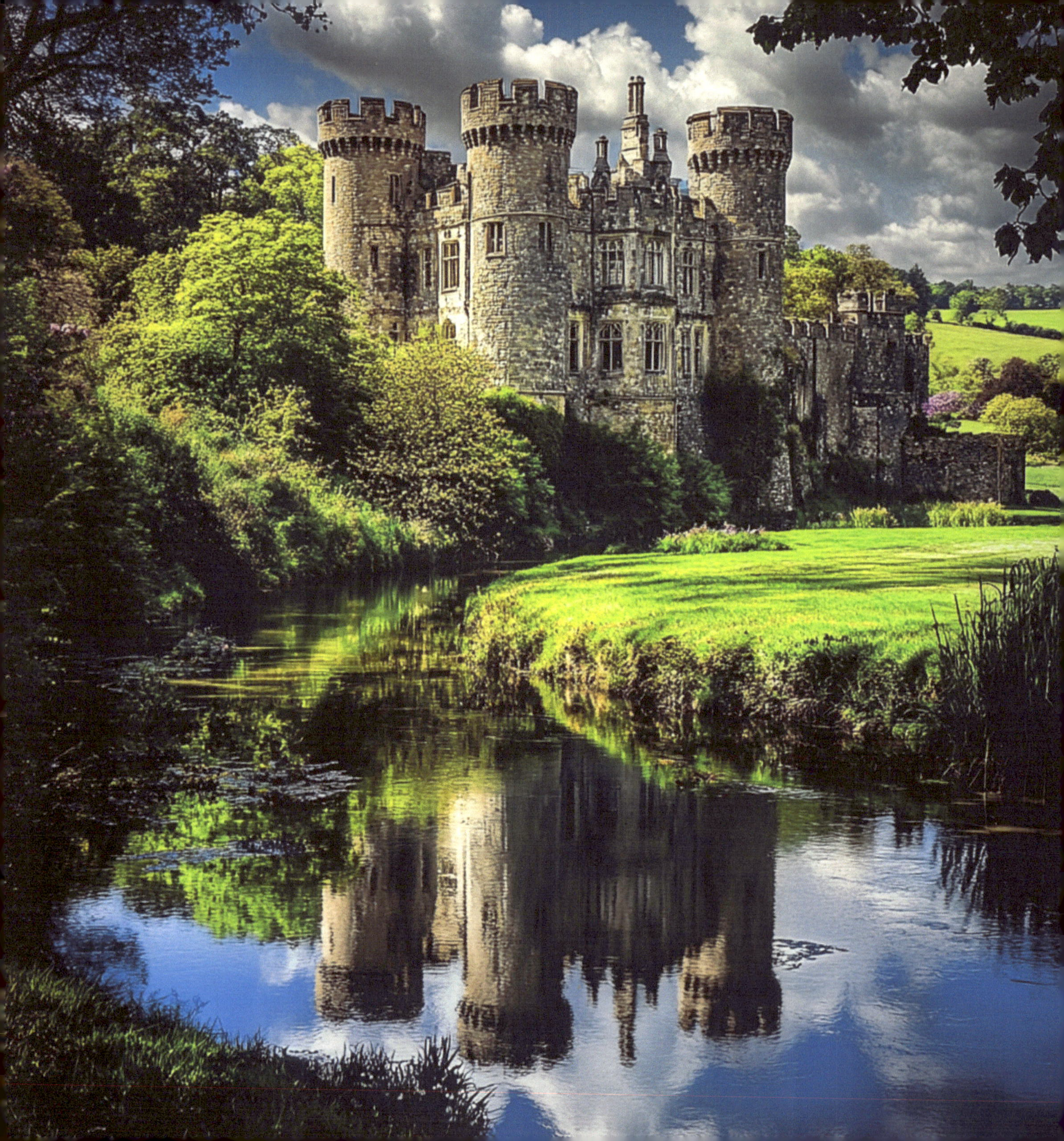

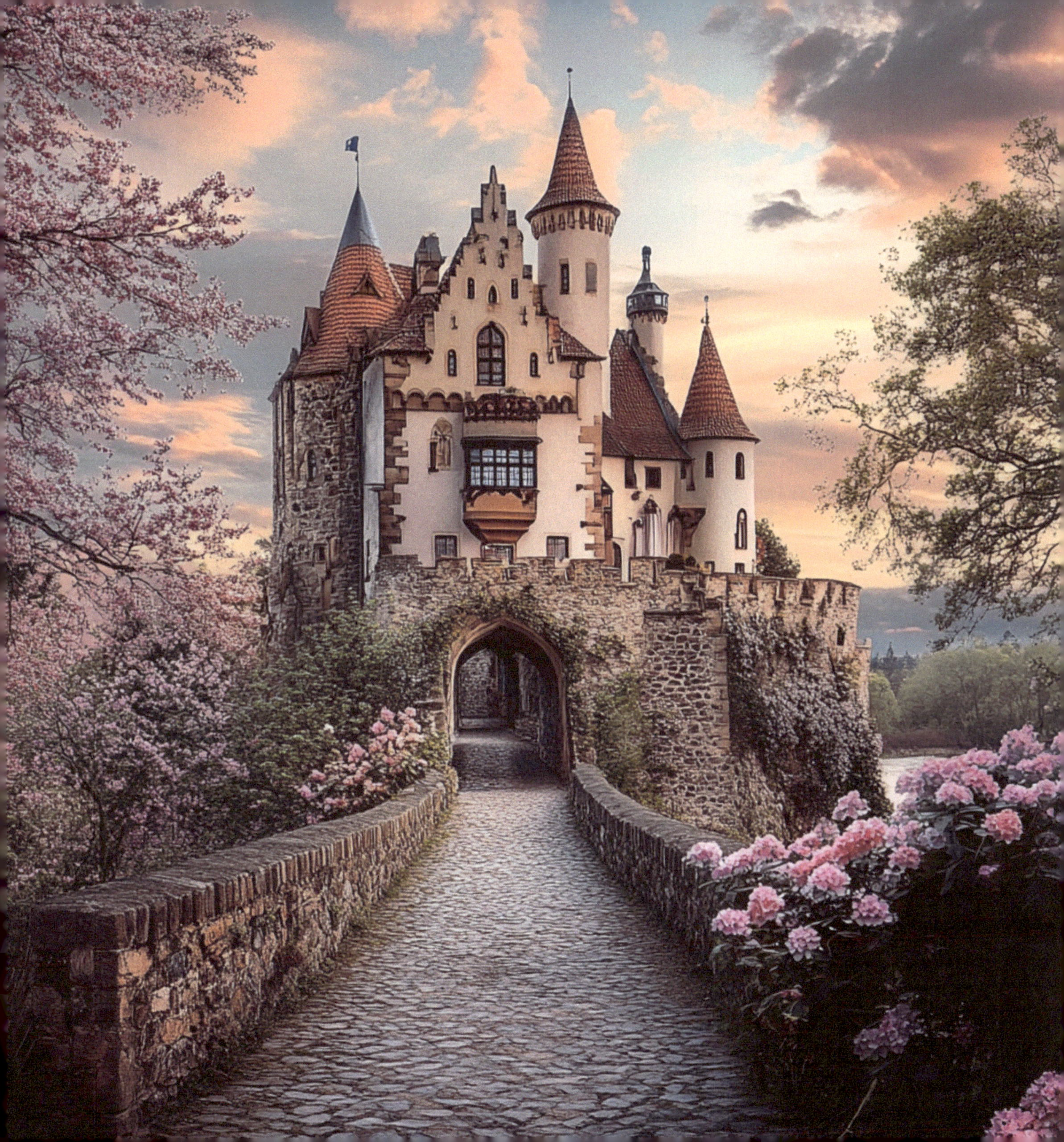

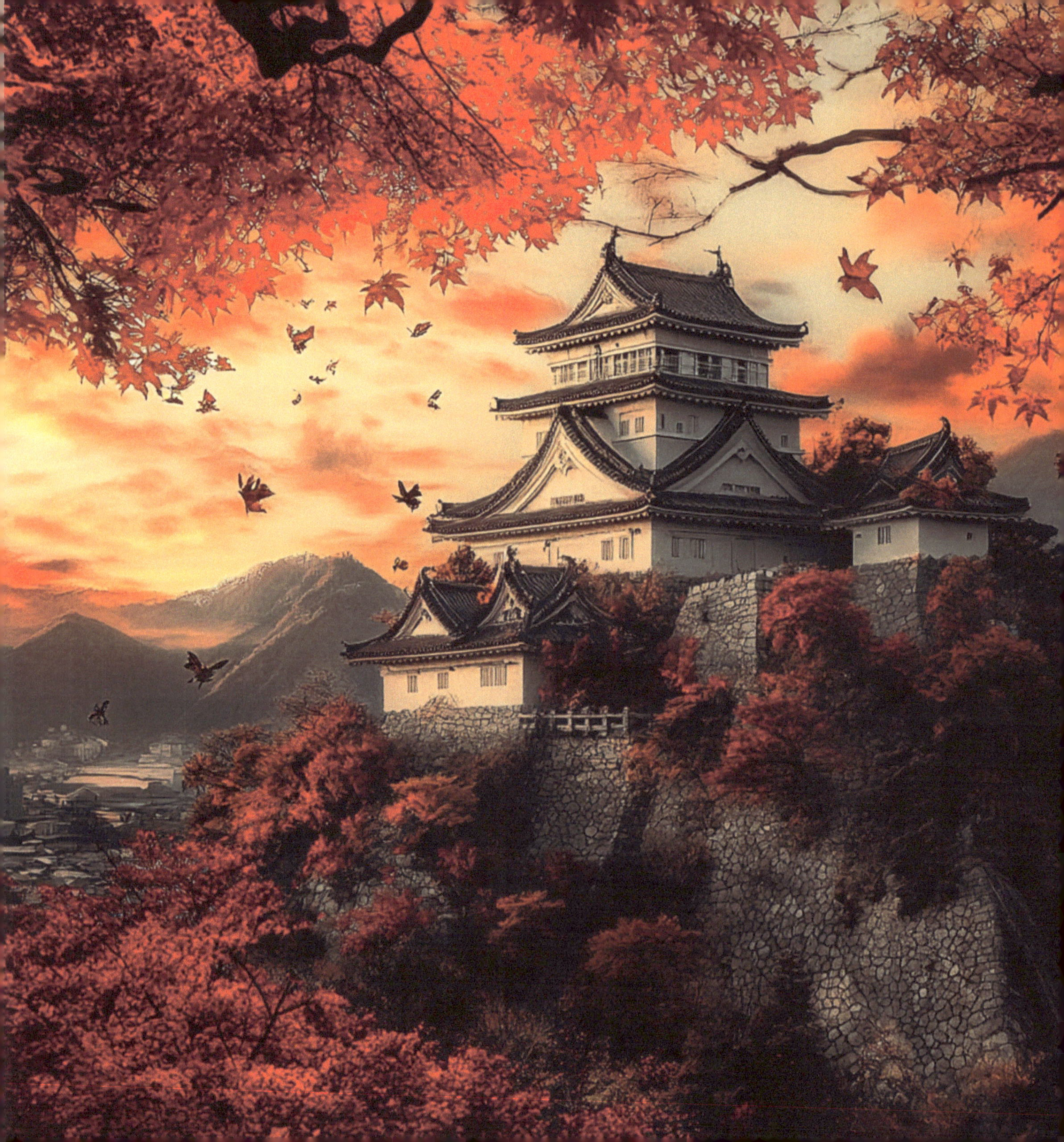

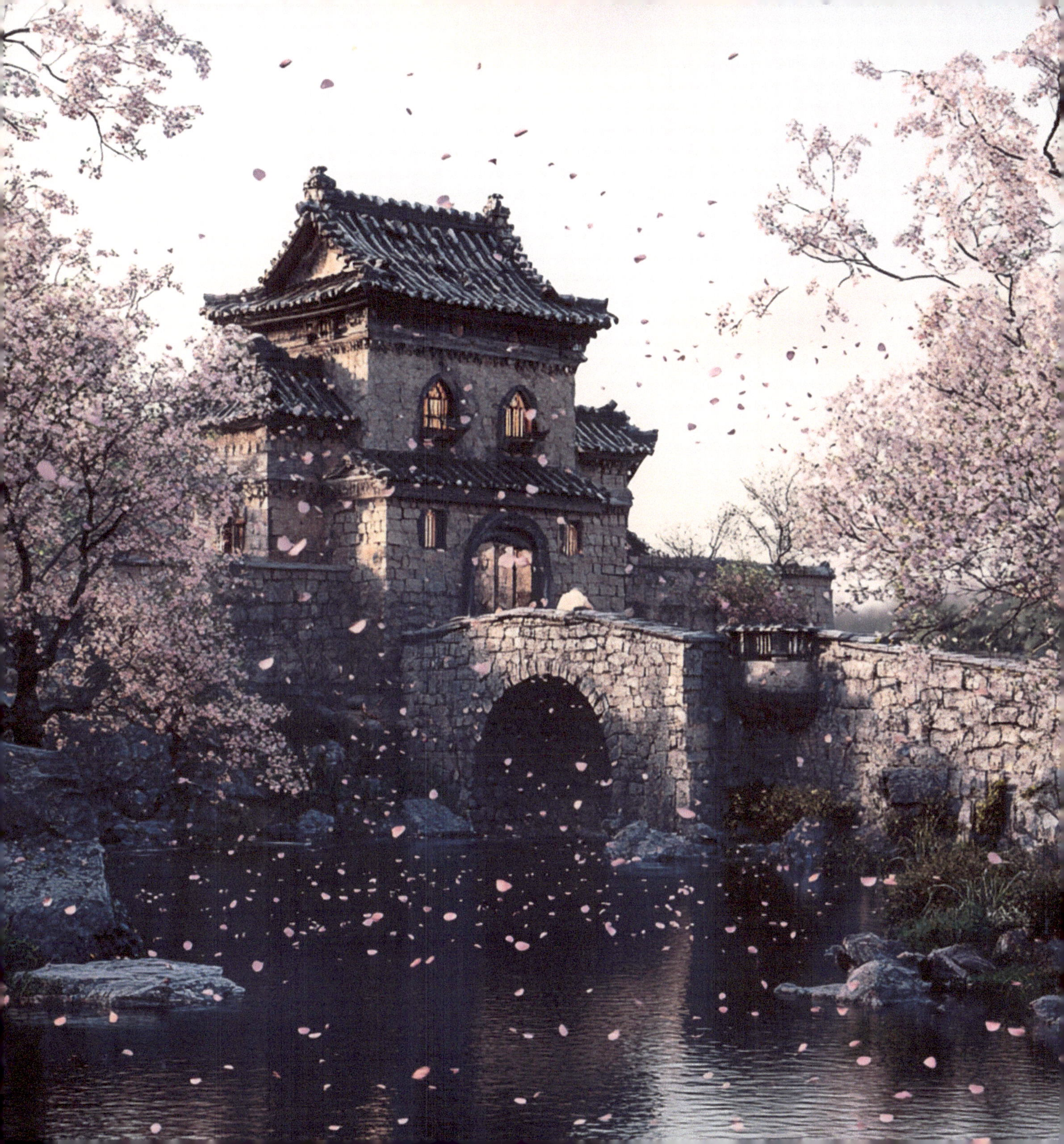

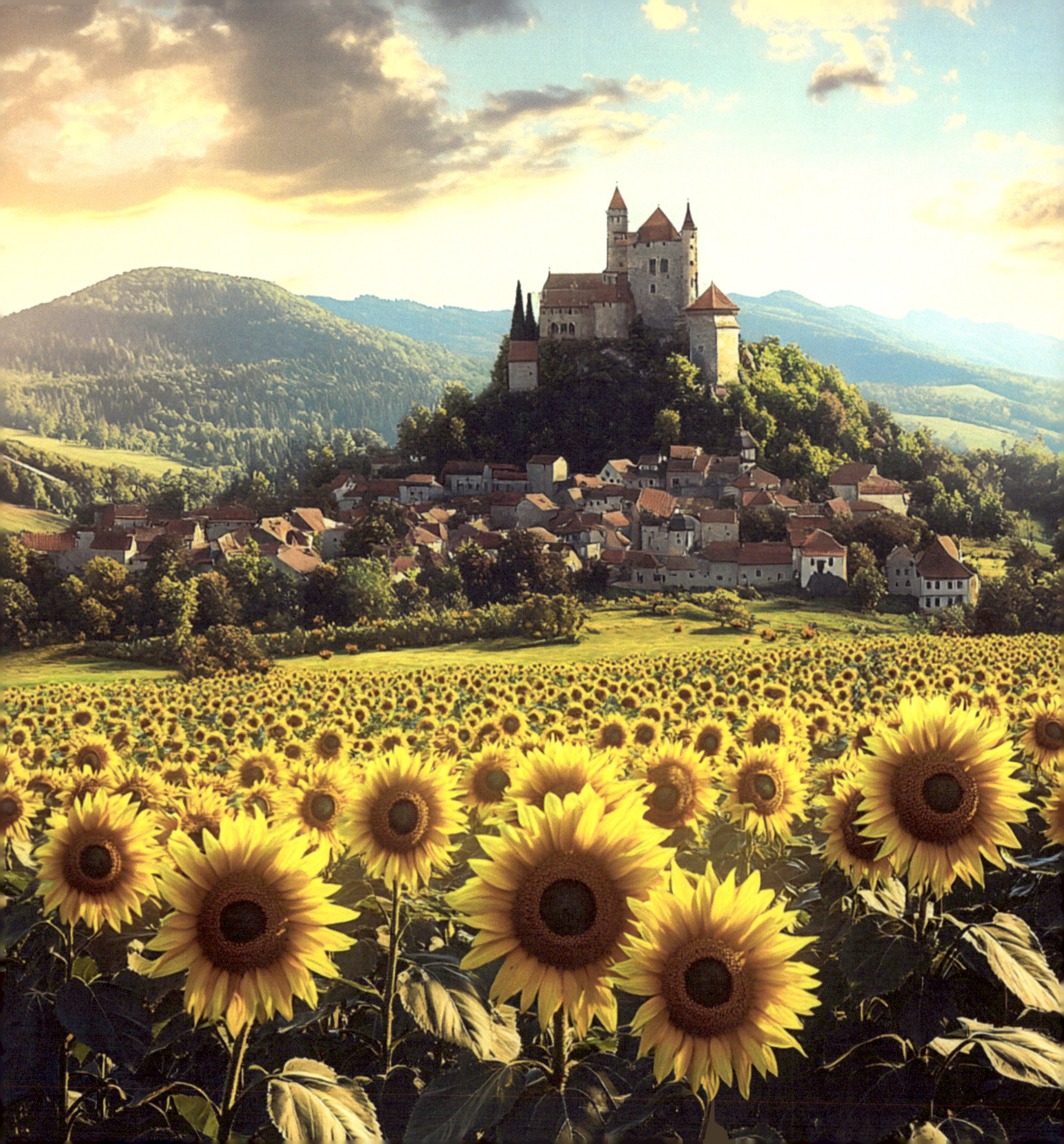

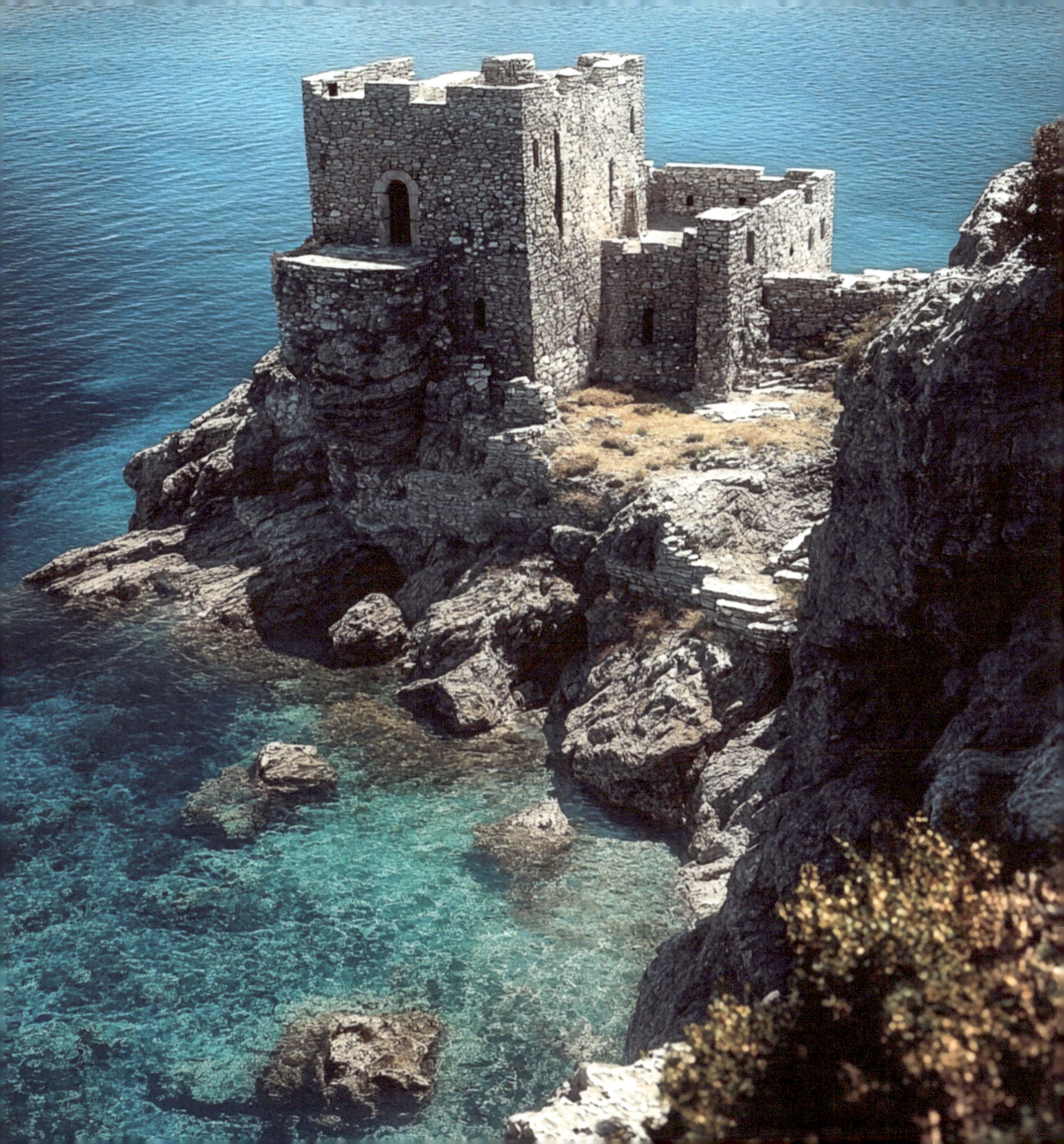

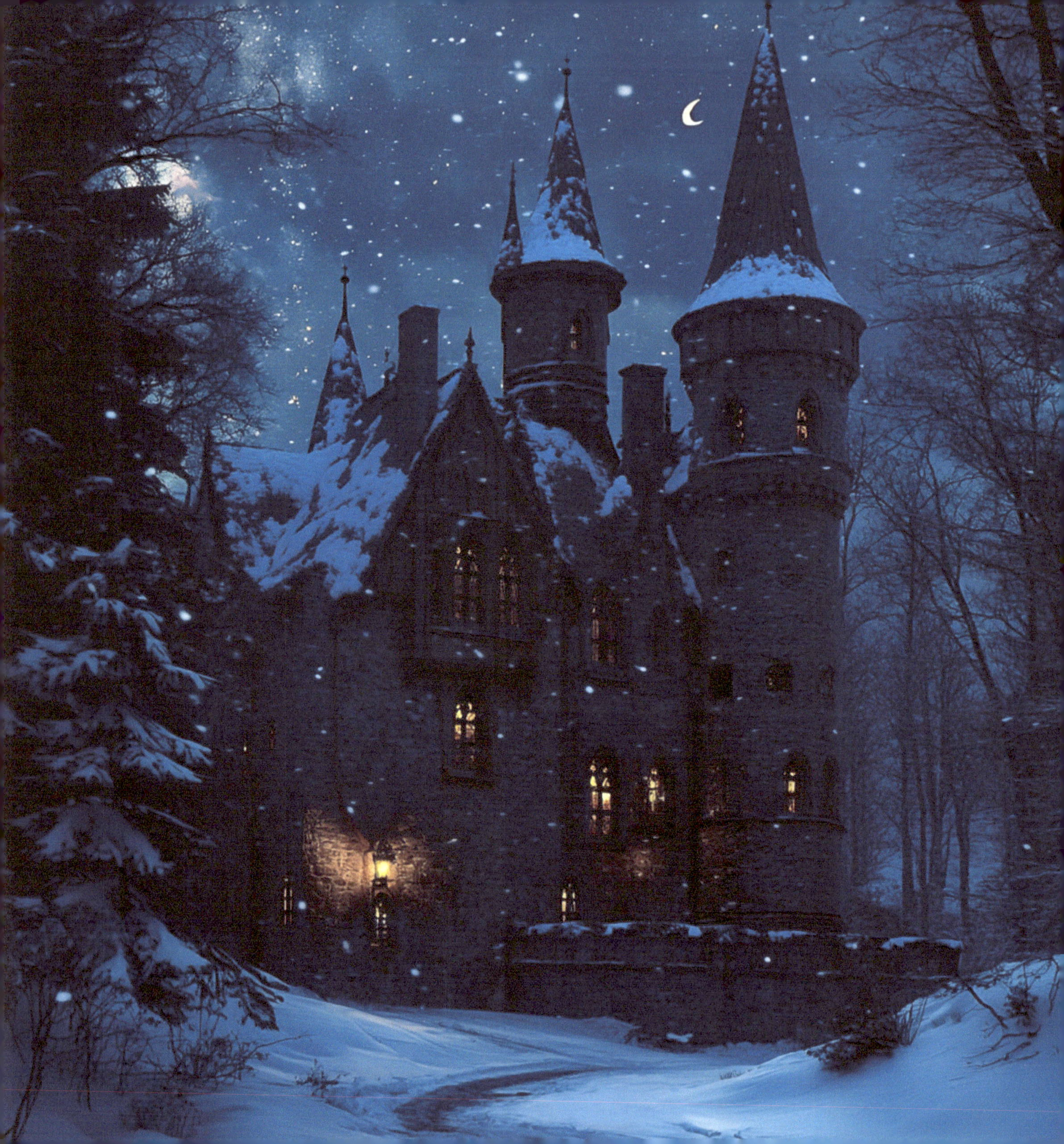

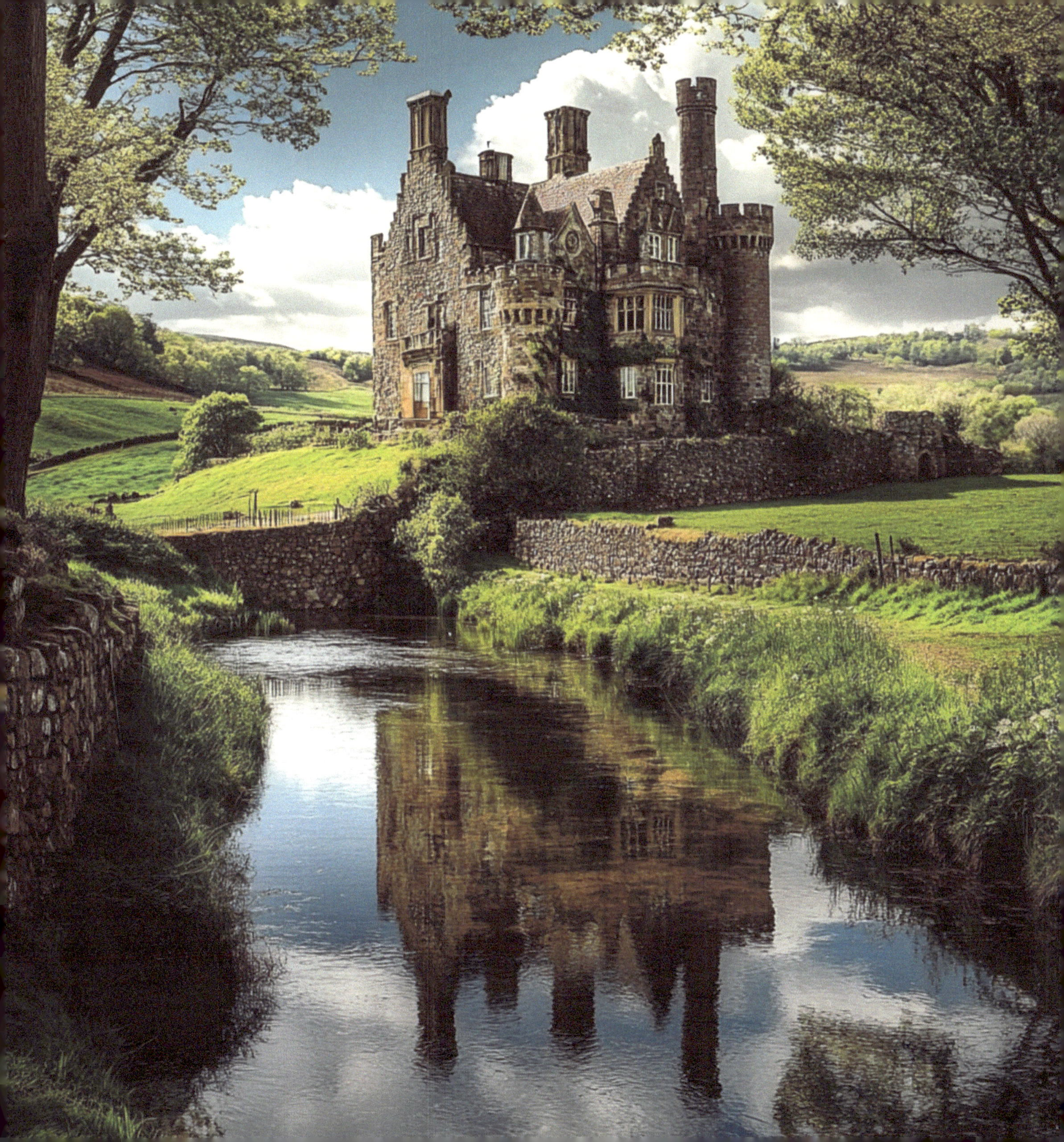

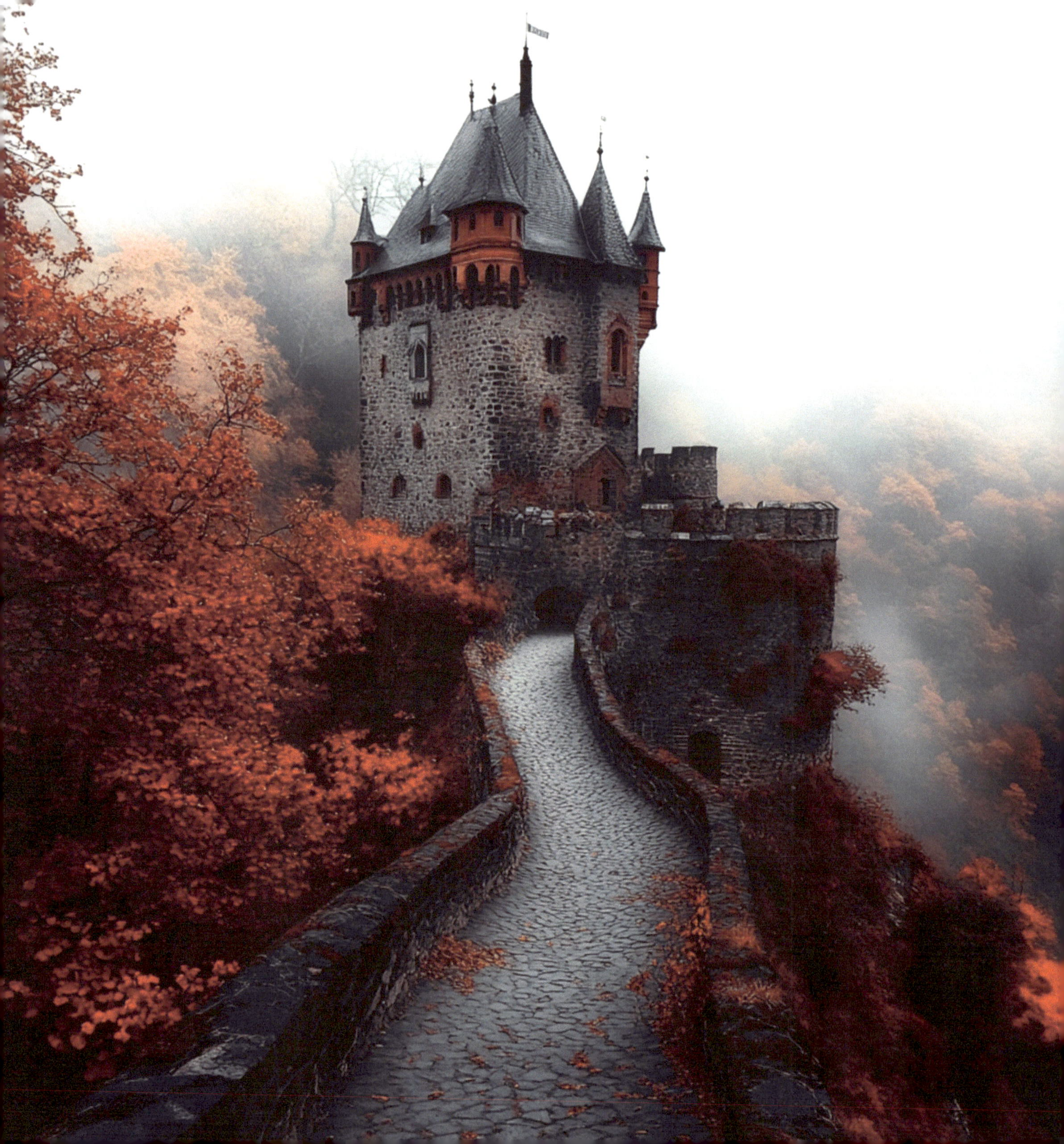

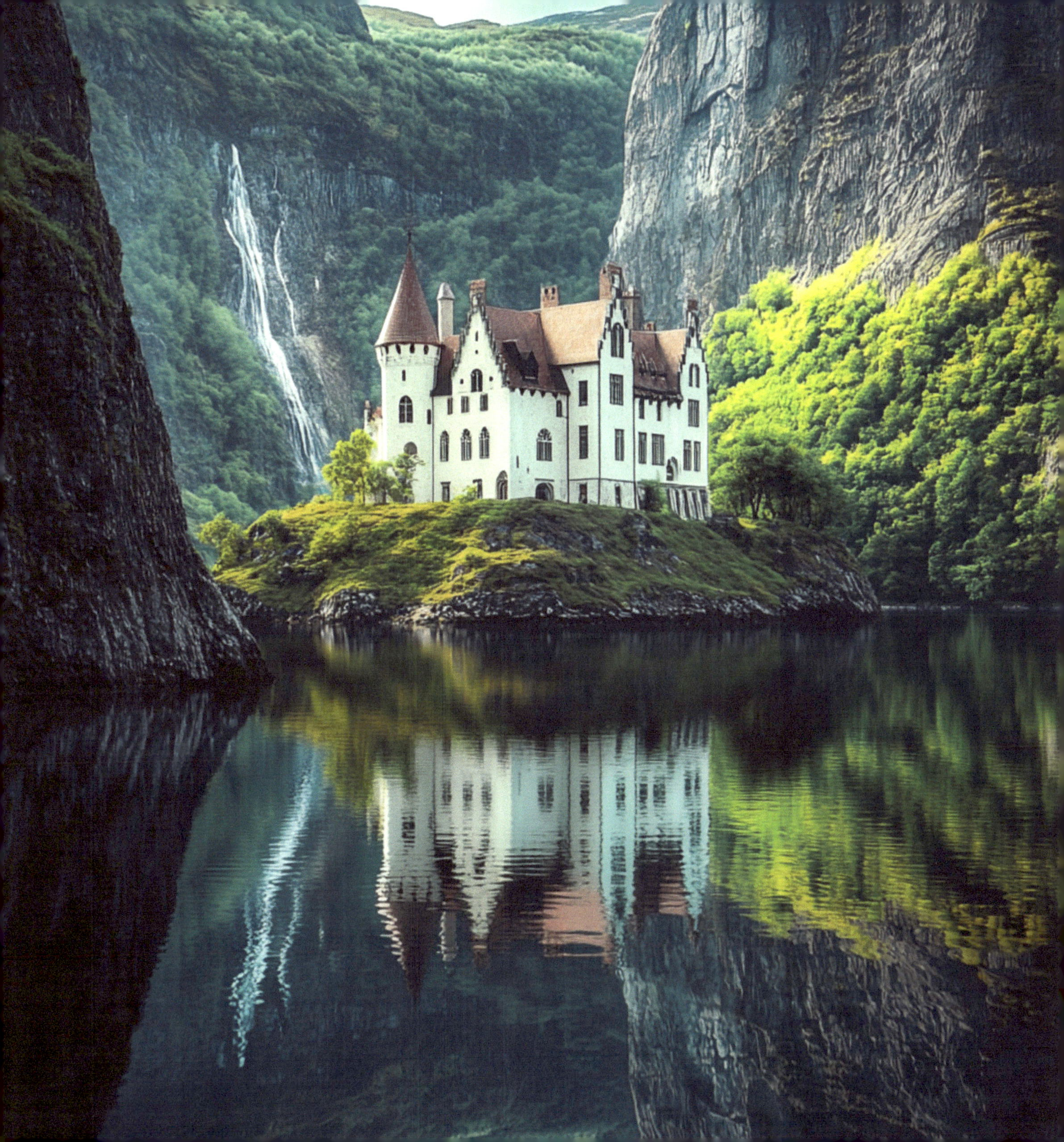

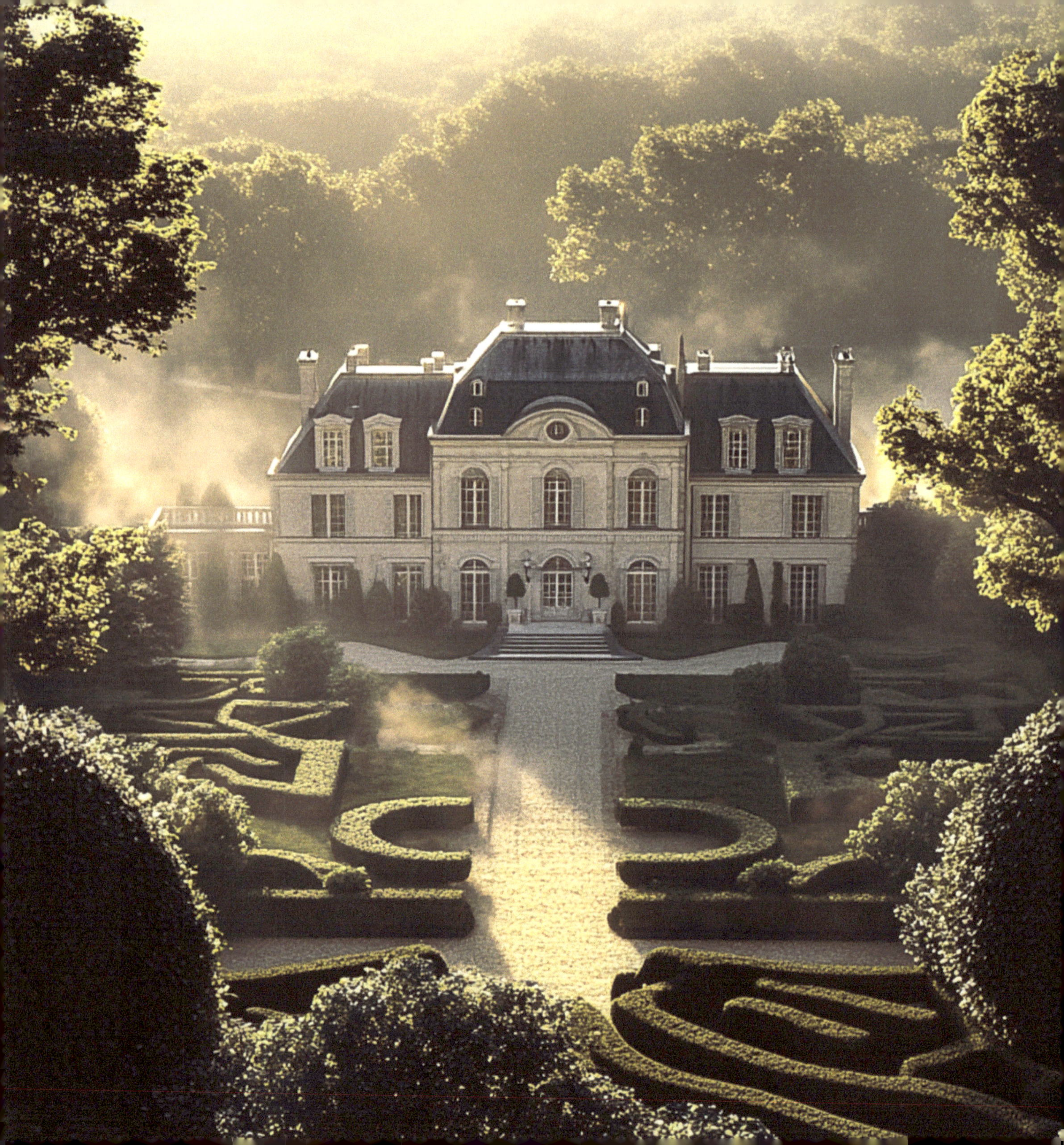

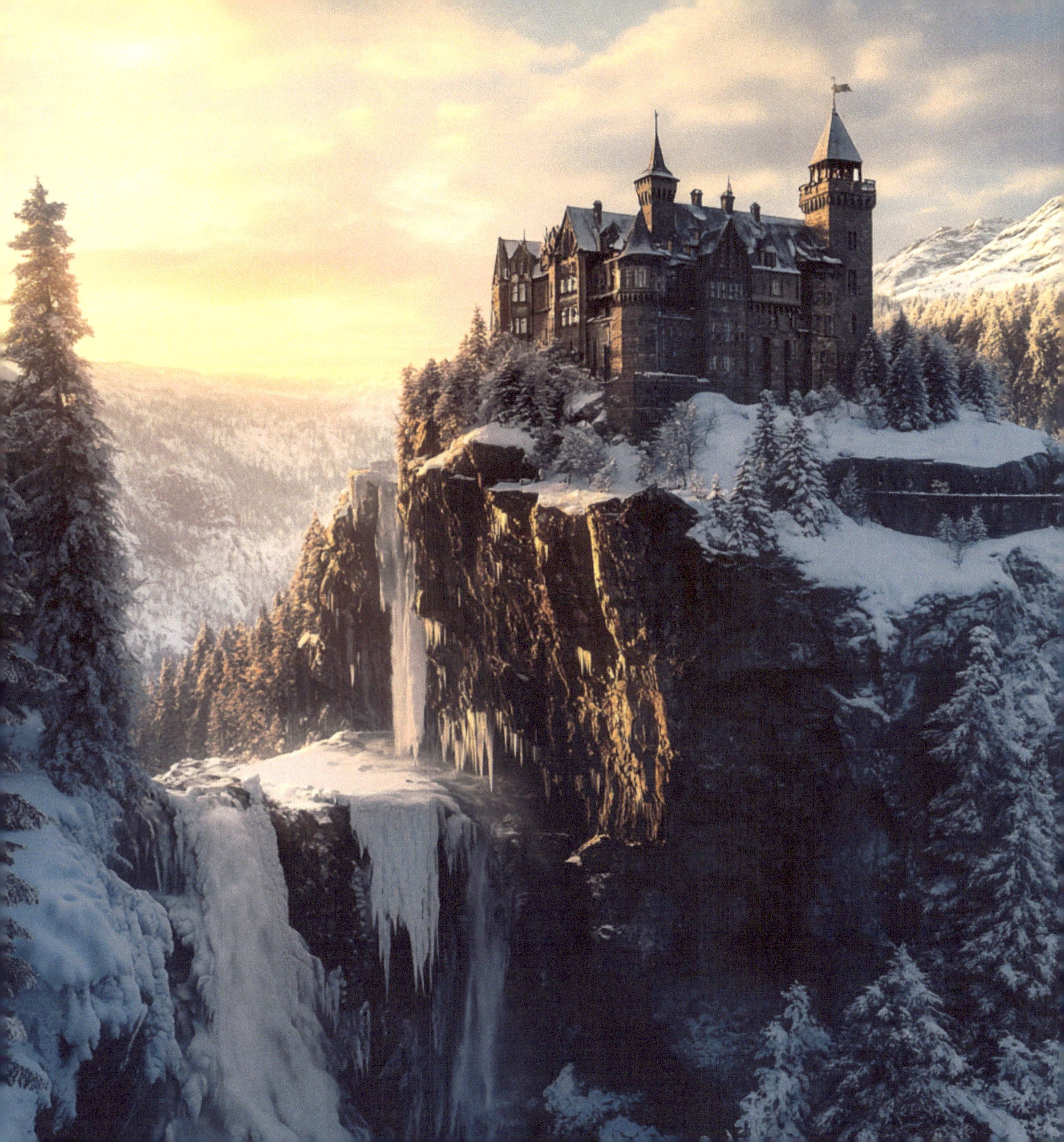

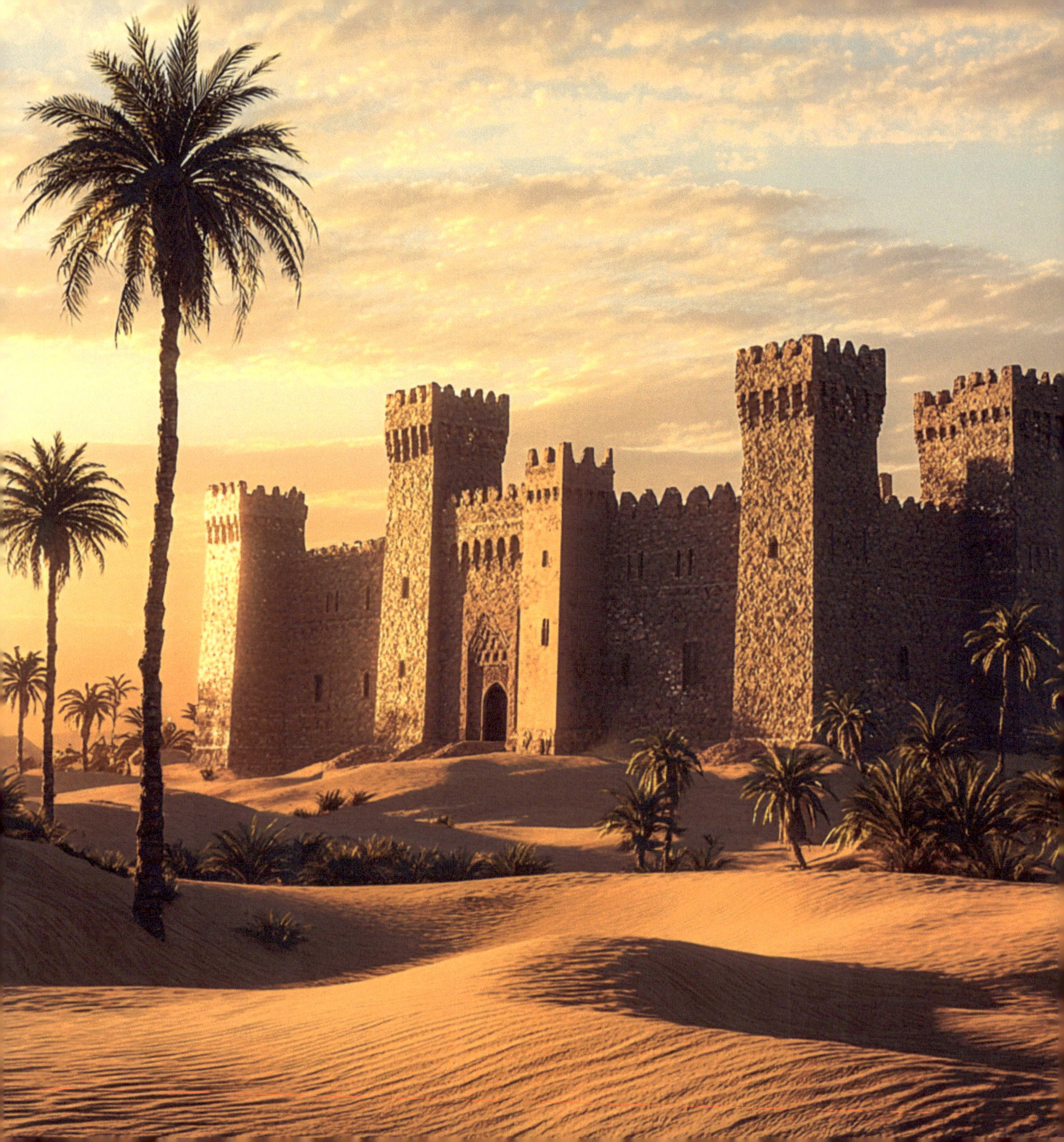

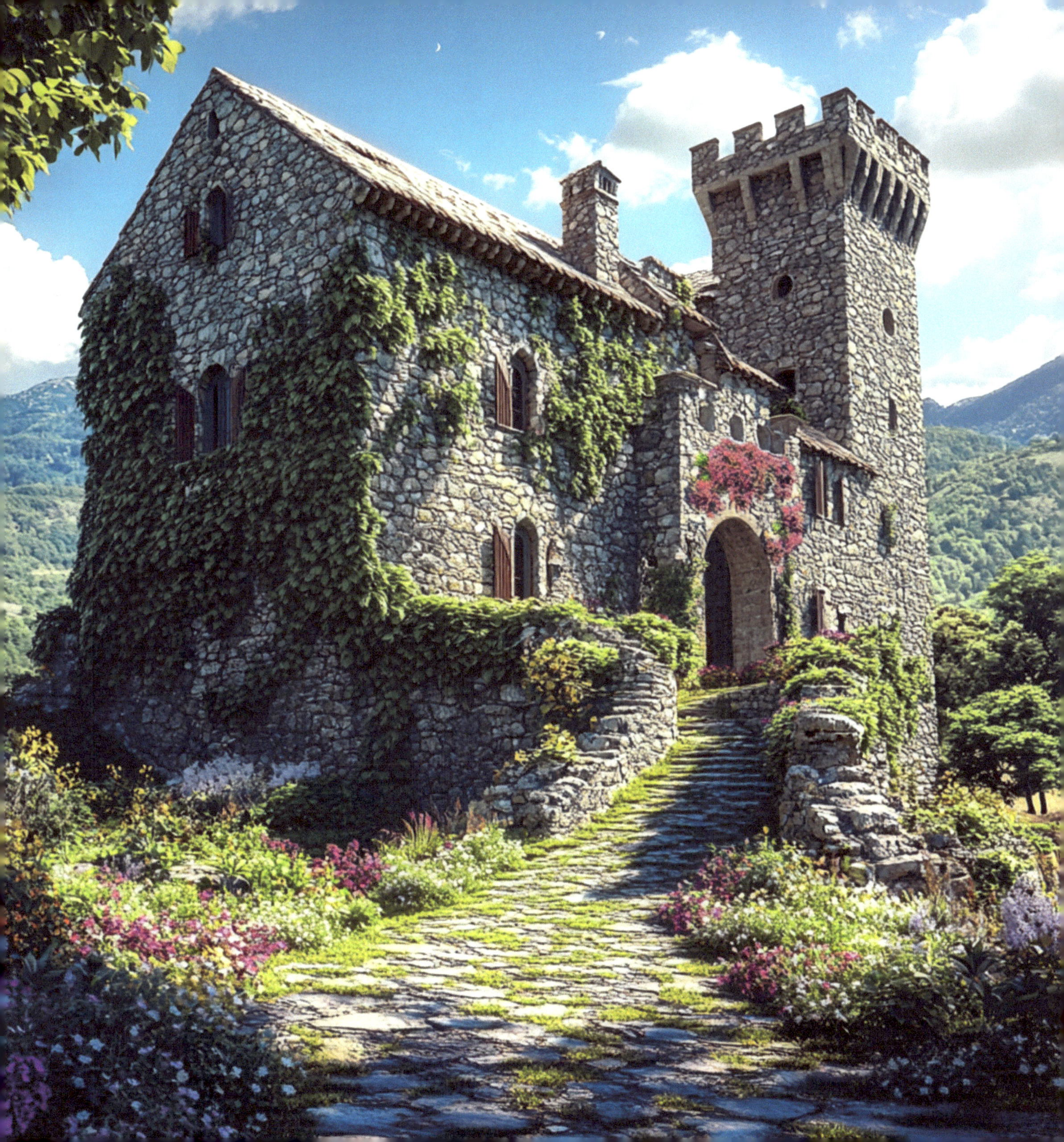

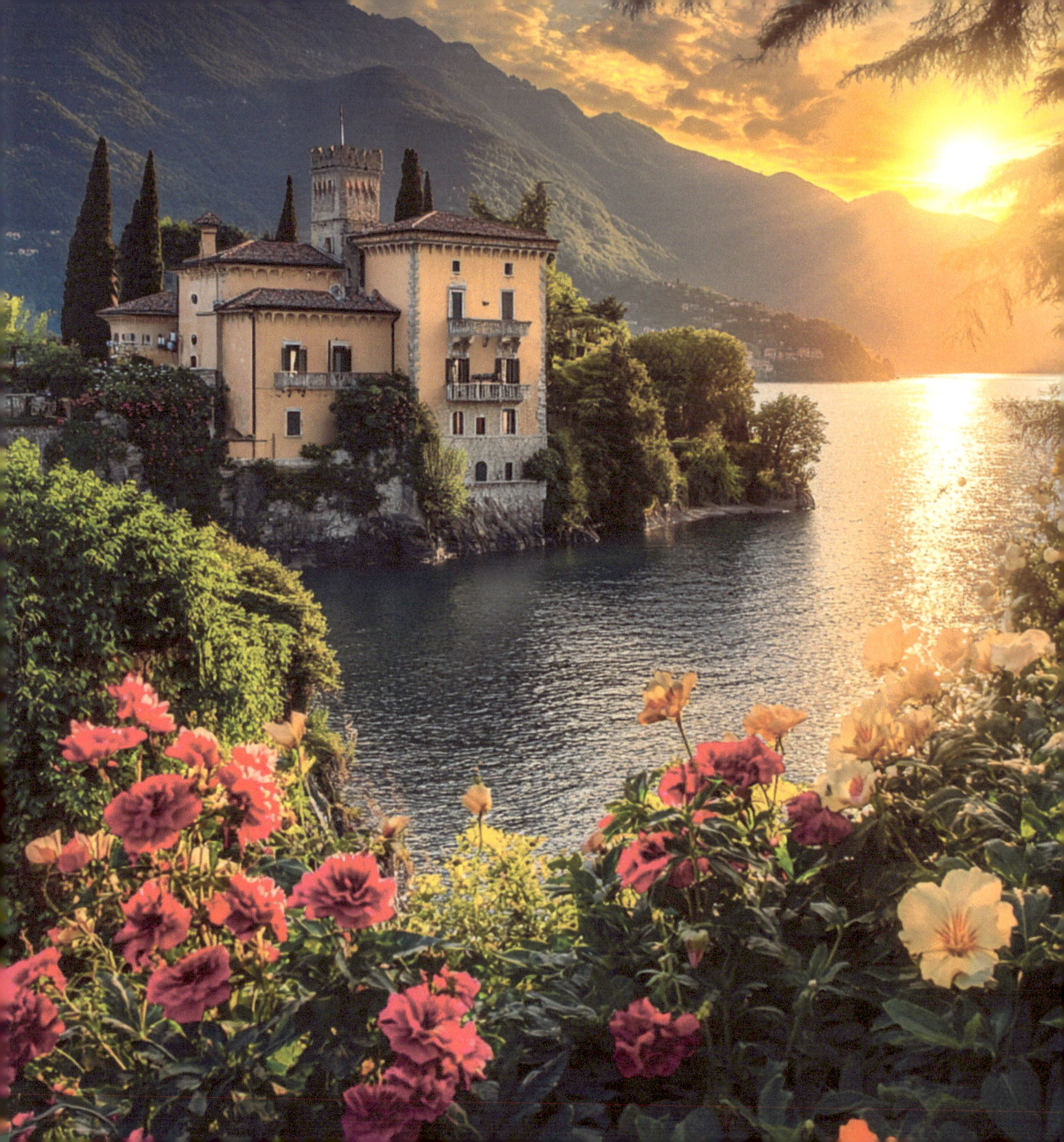

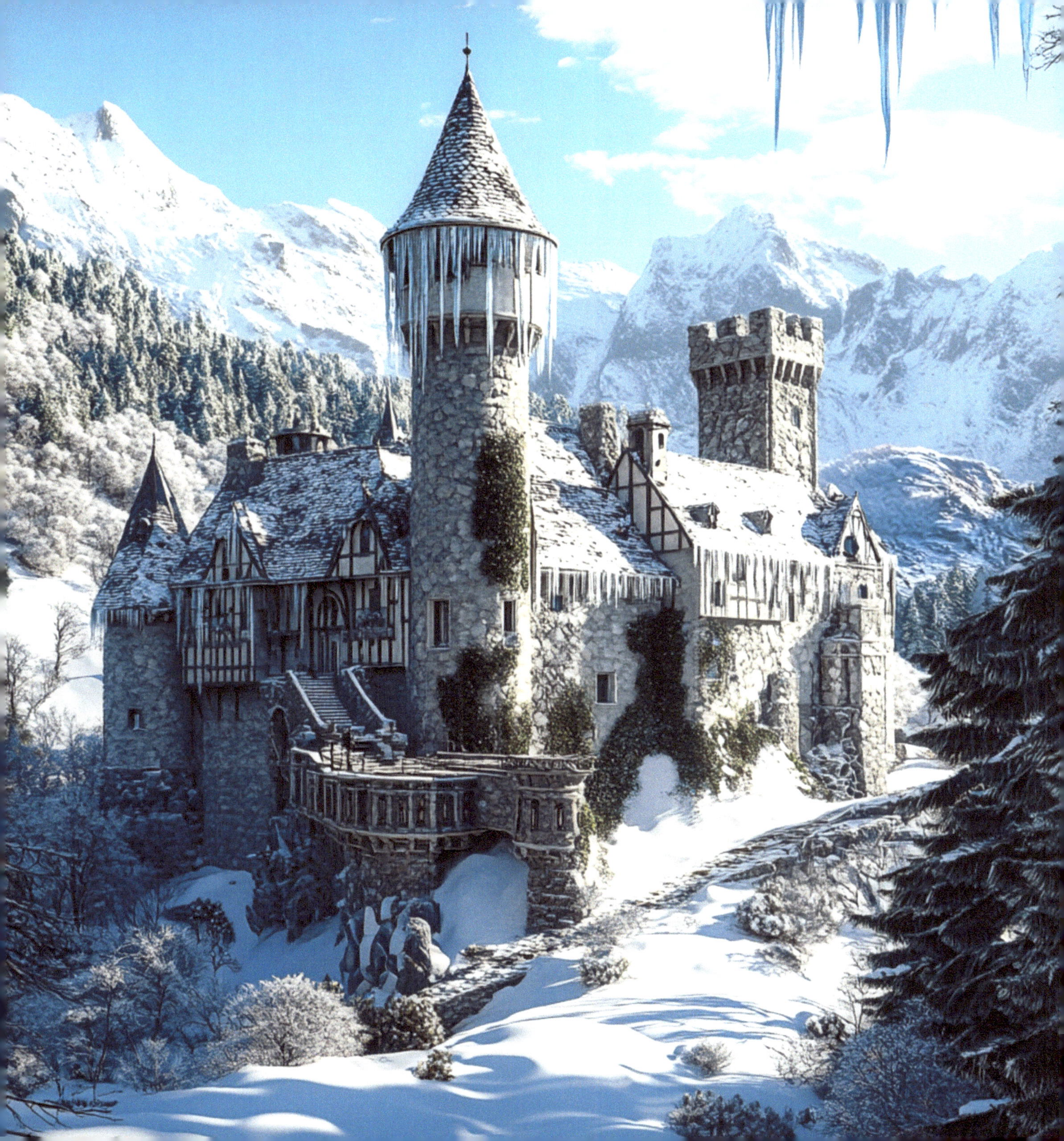

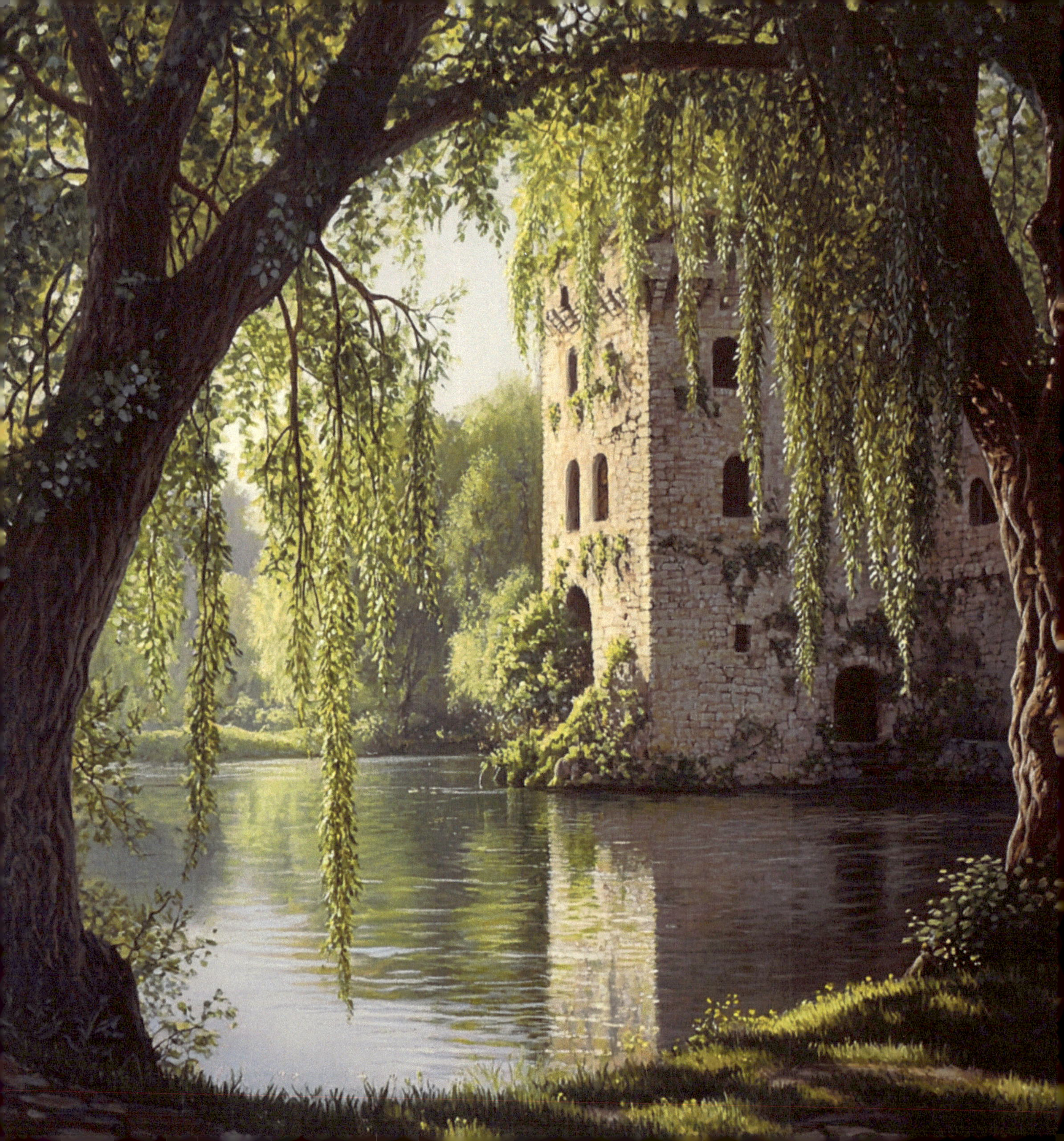

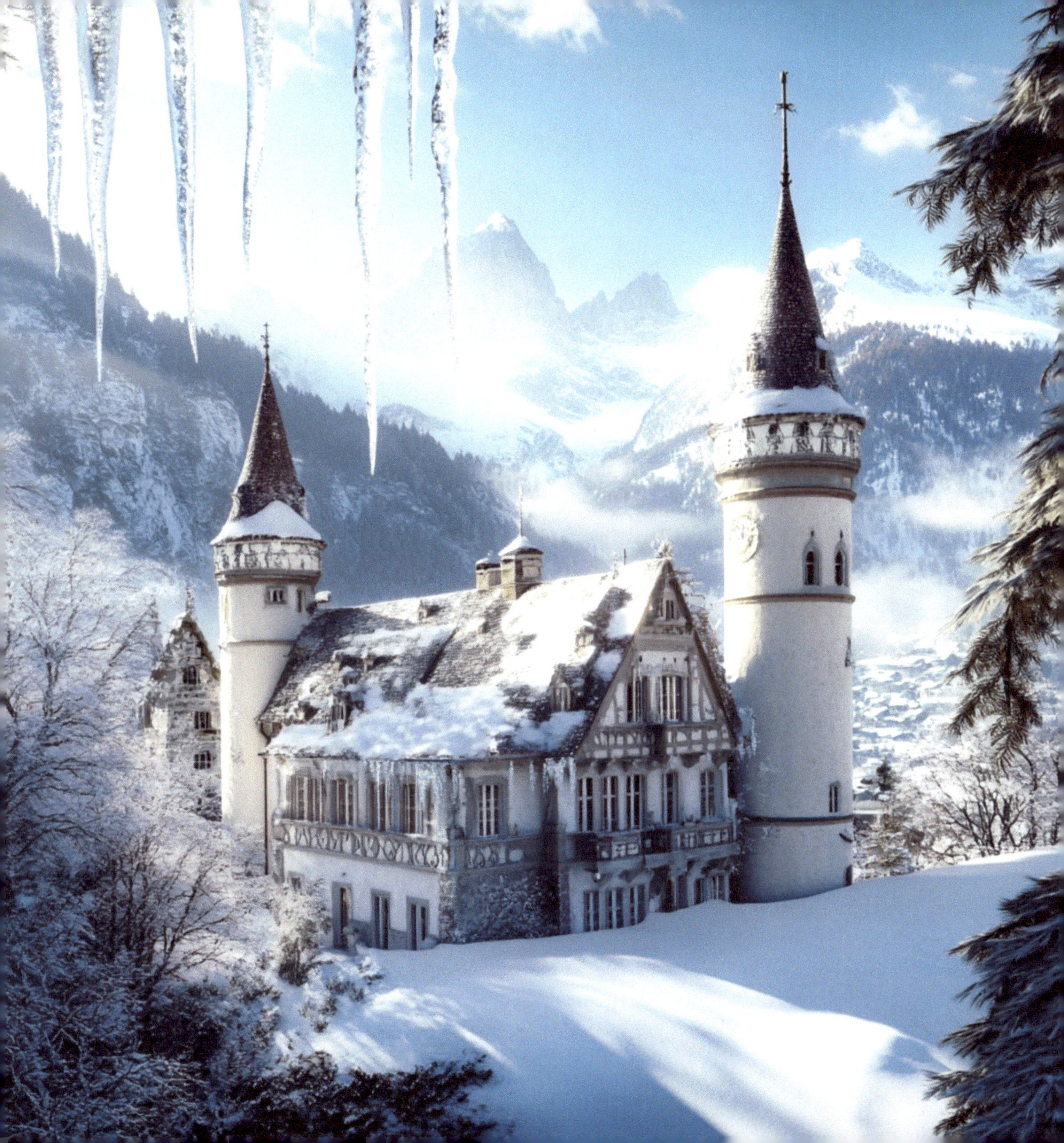

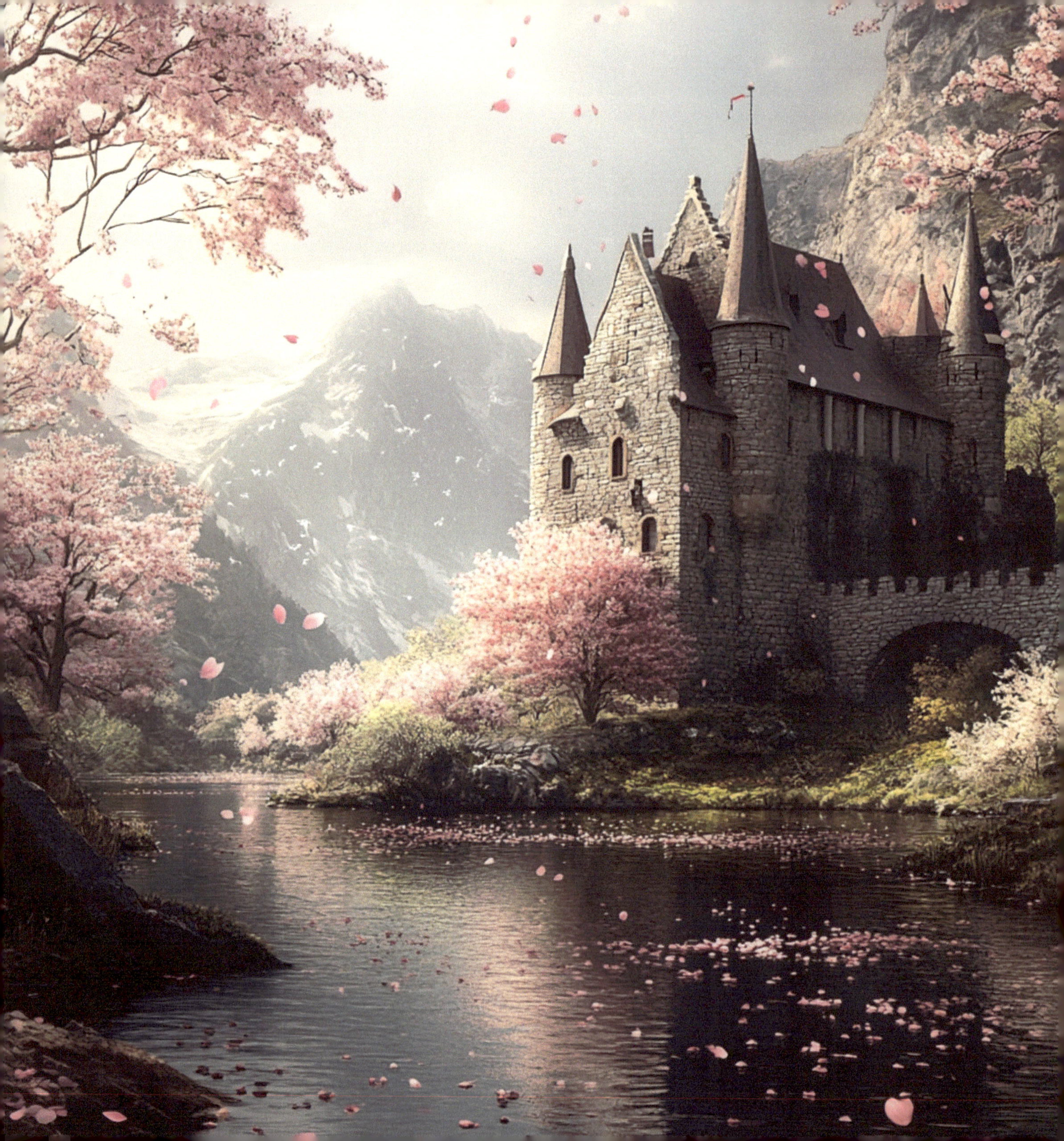

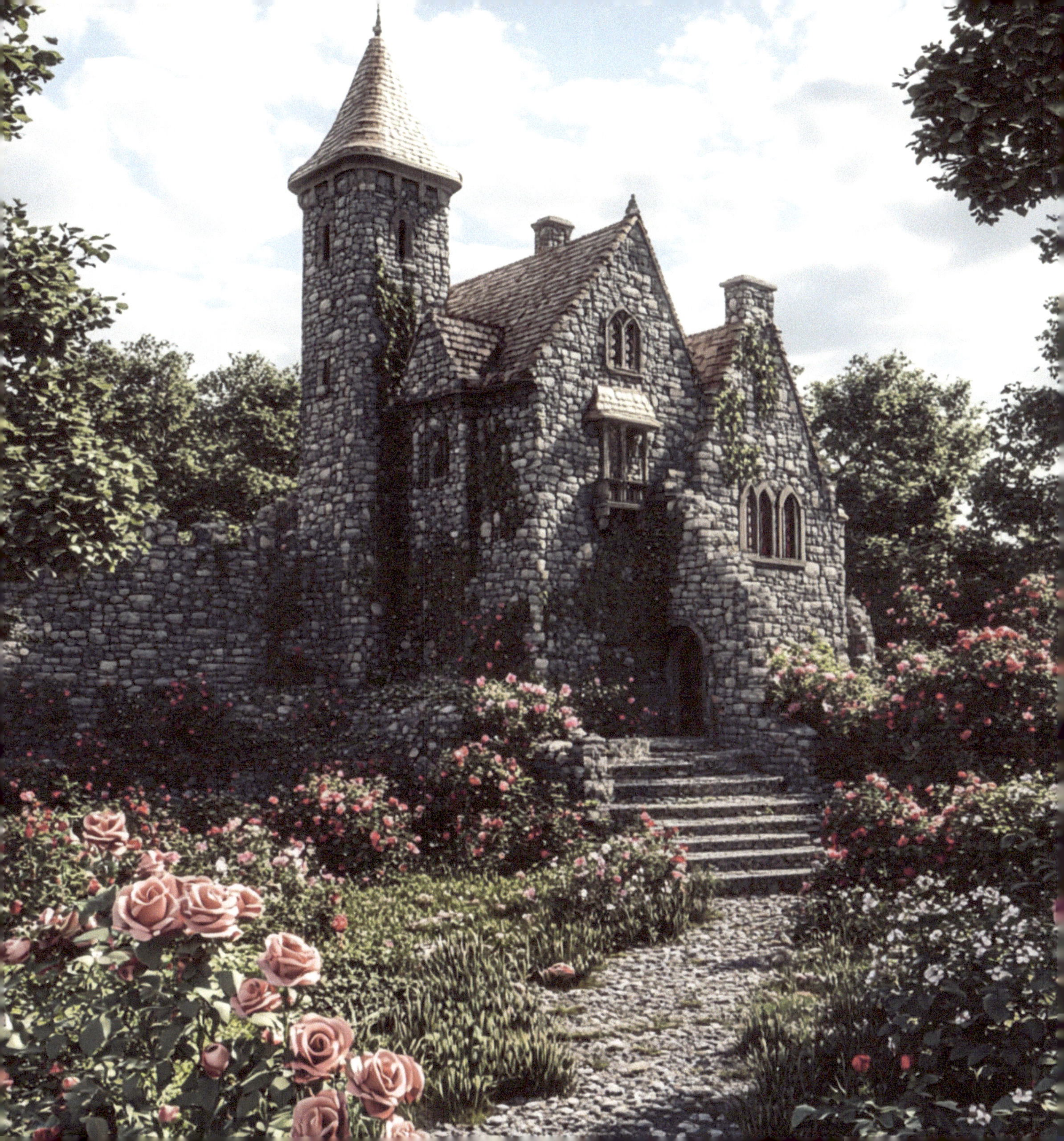

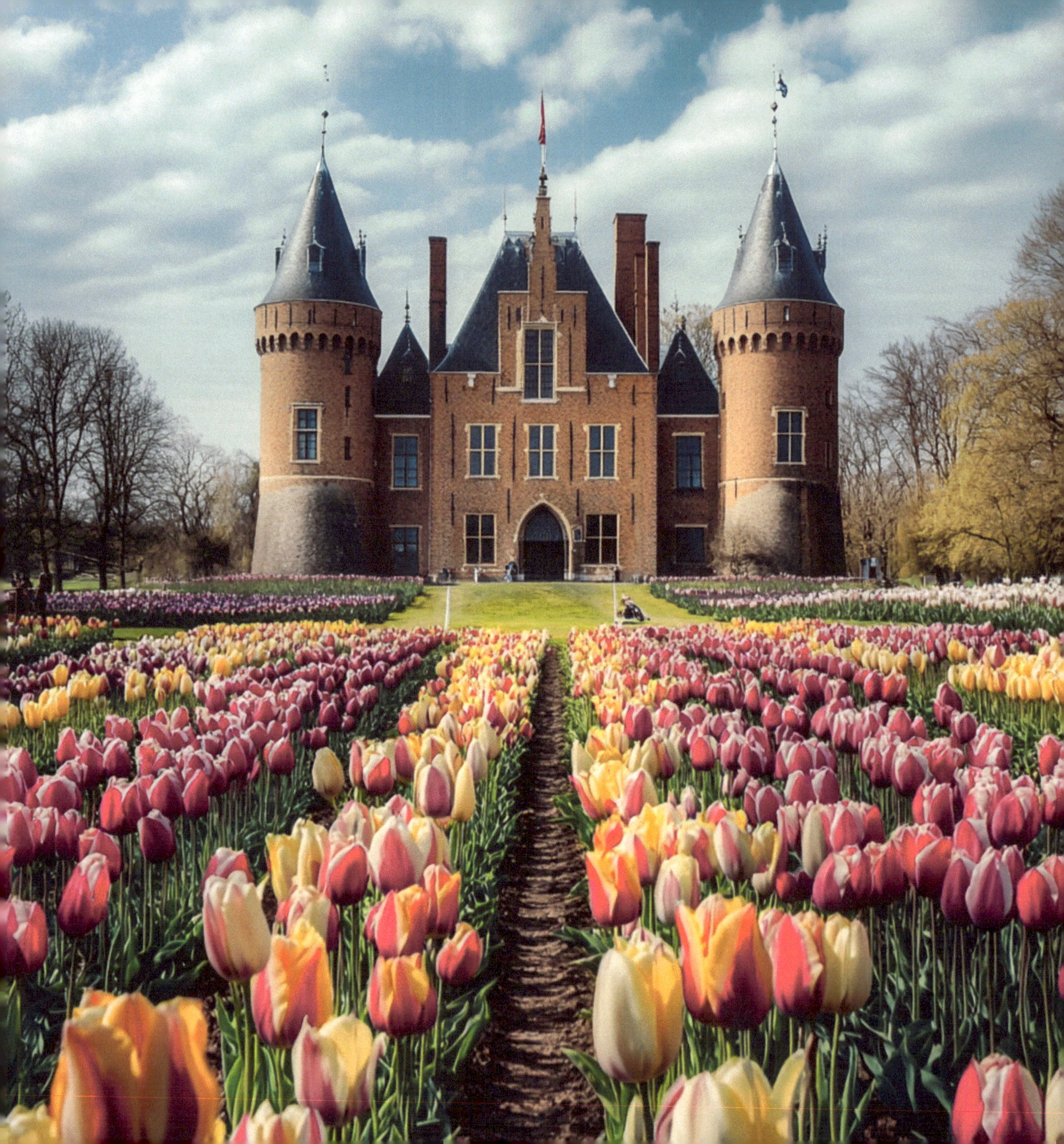

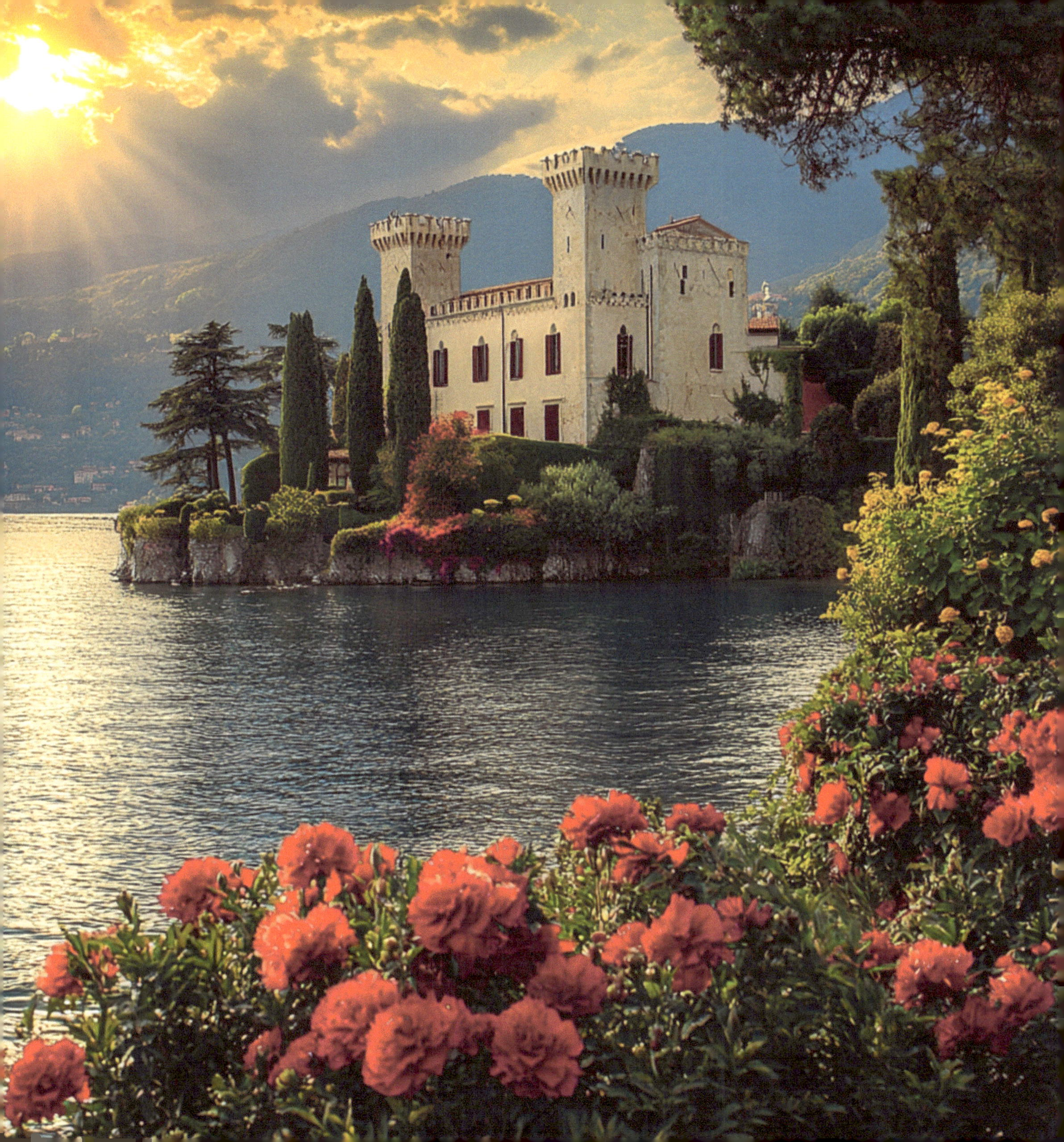

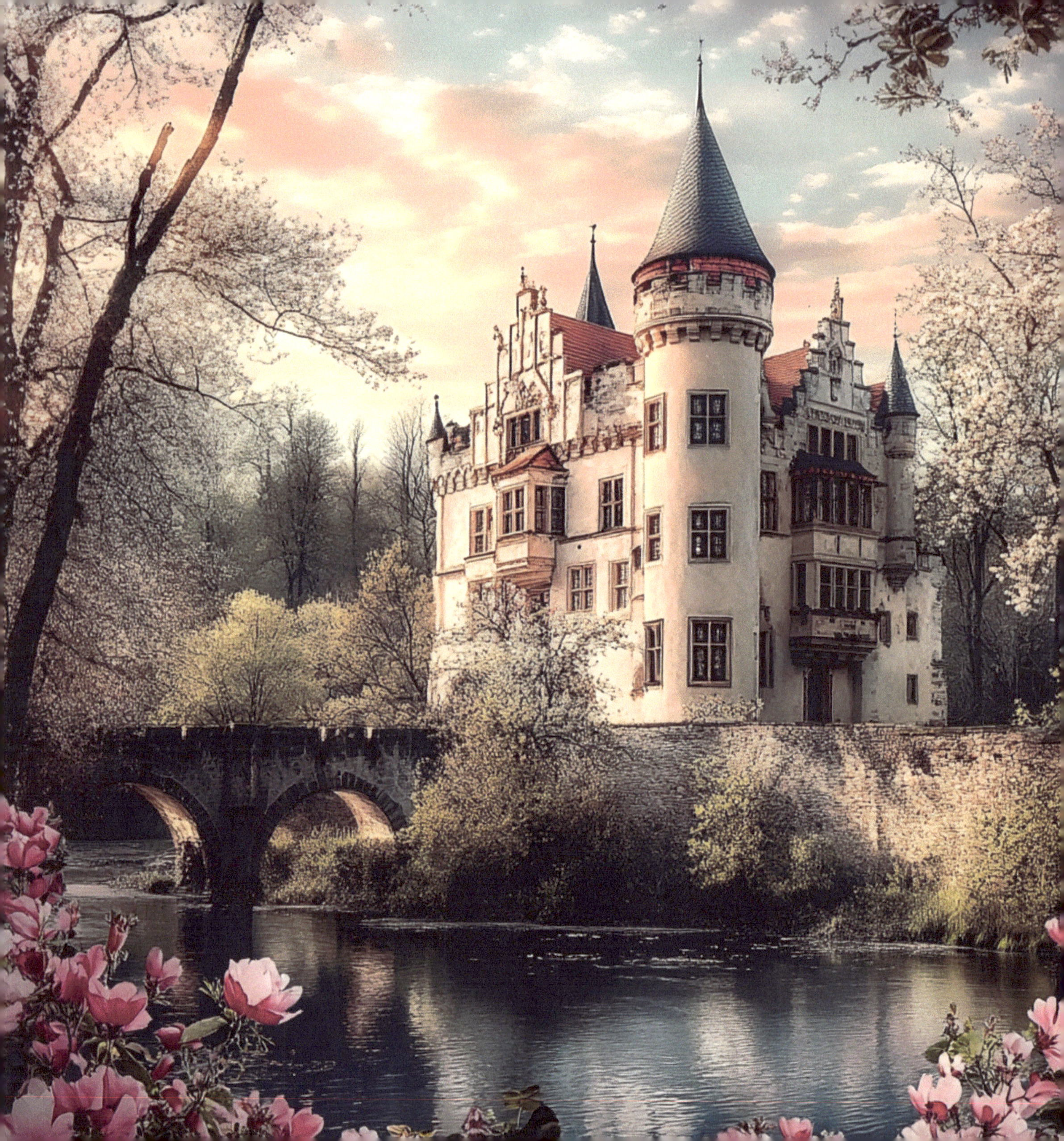

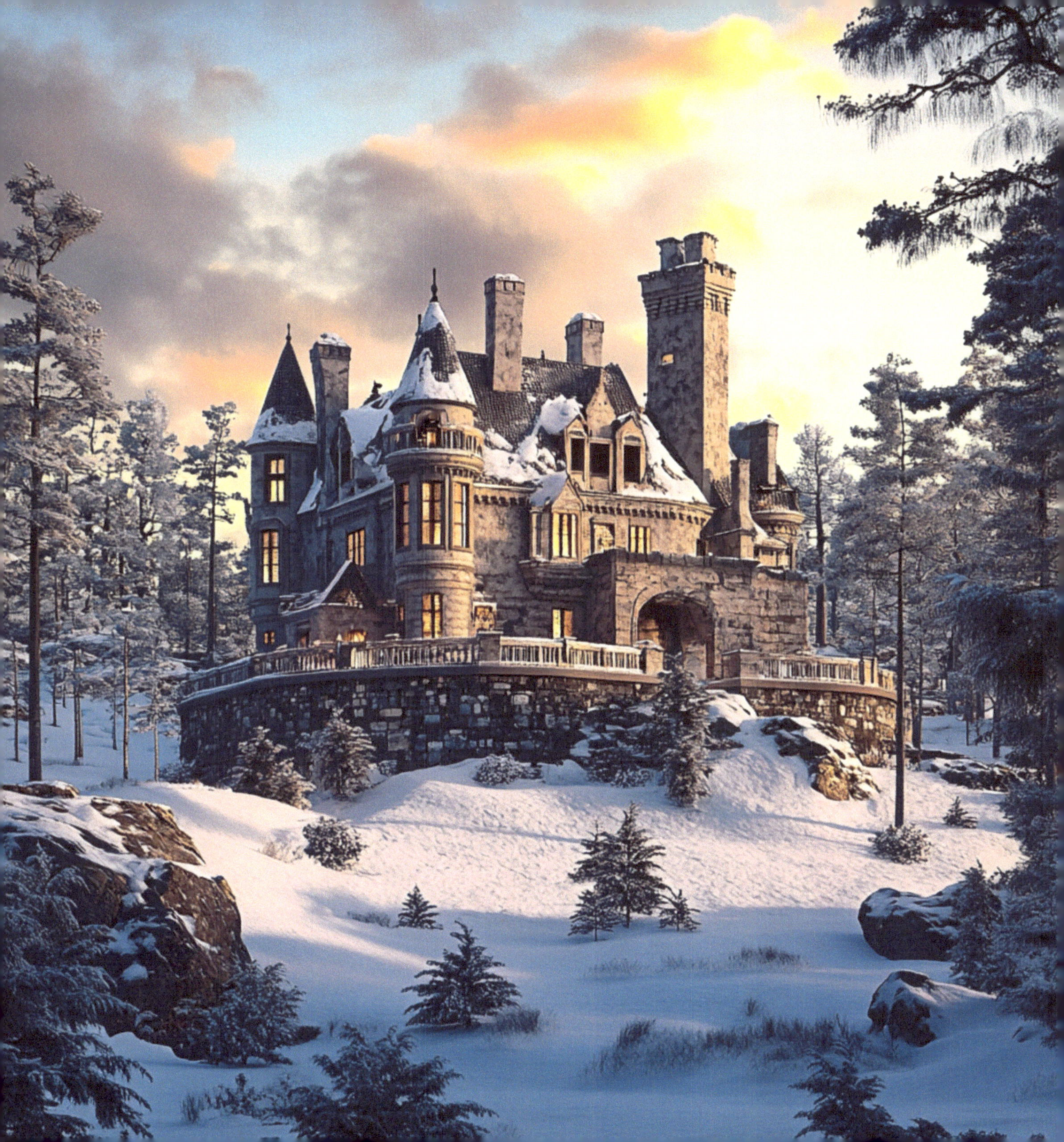

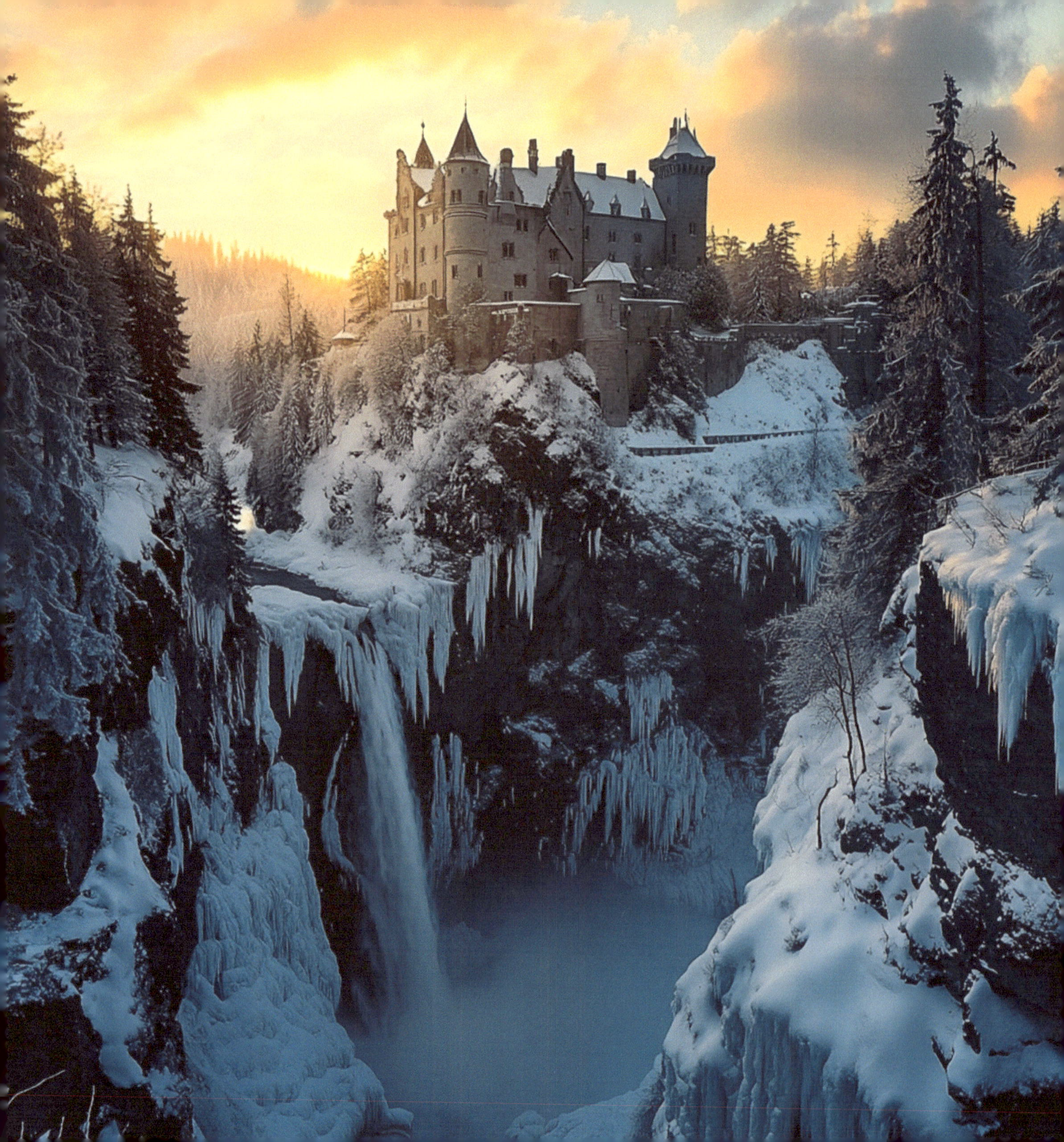

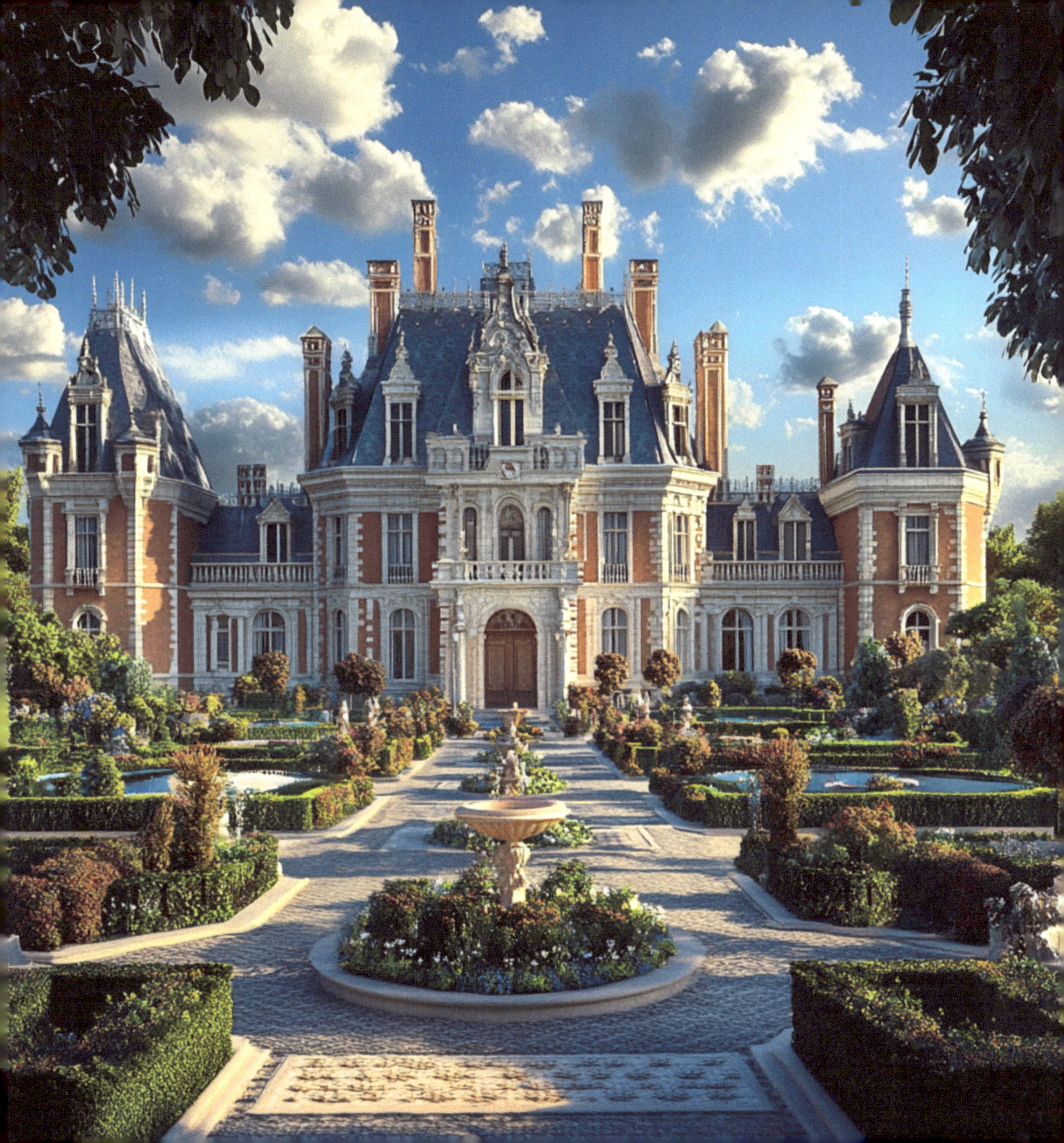

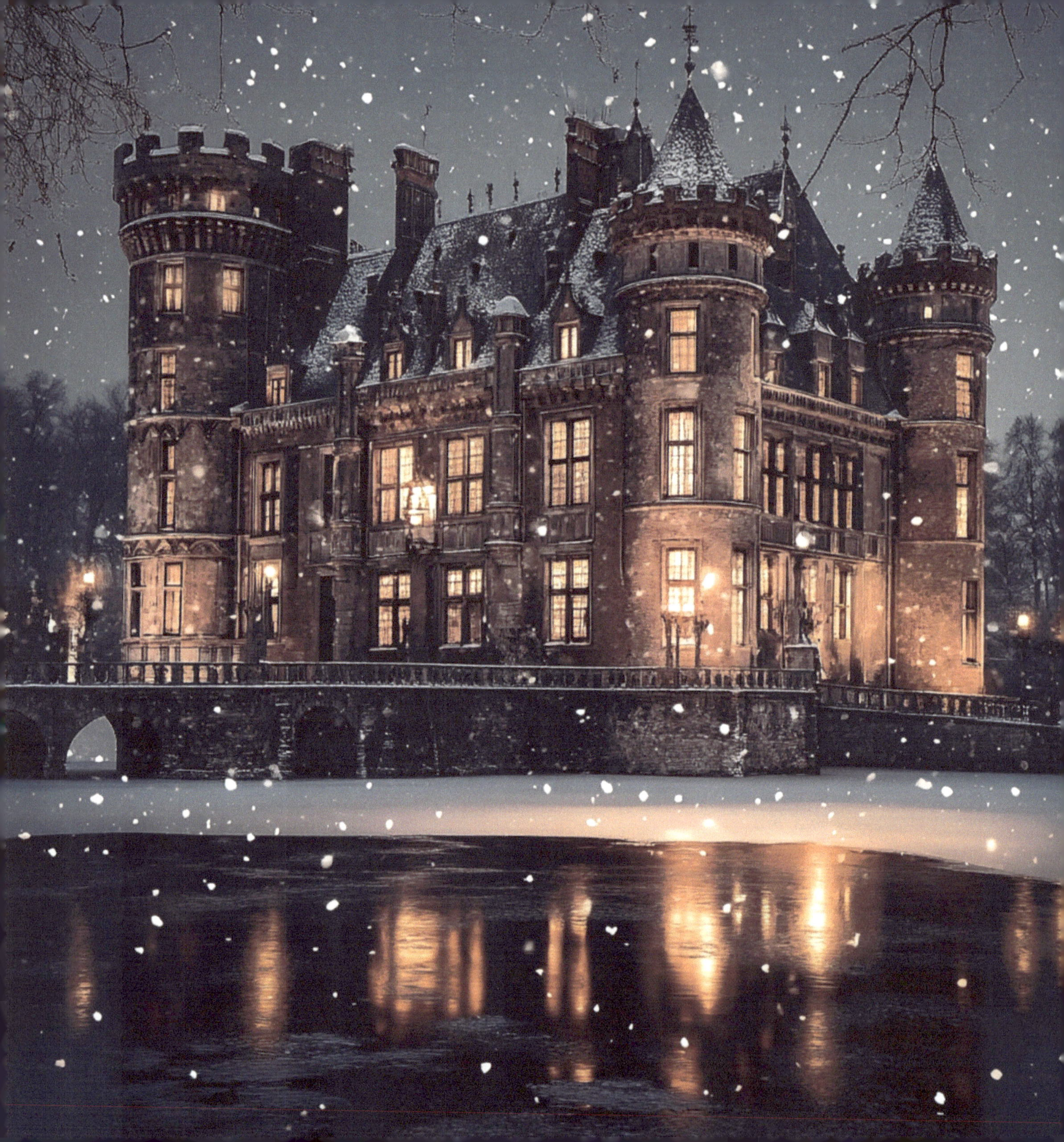

Other Books From Raeka Harding

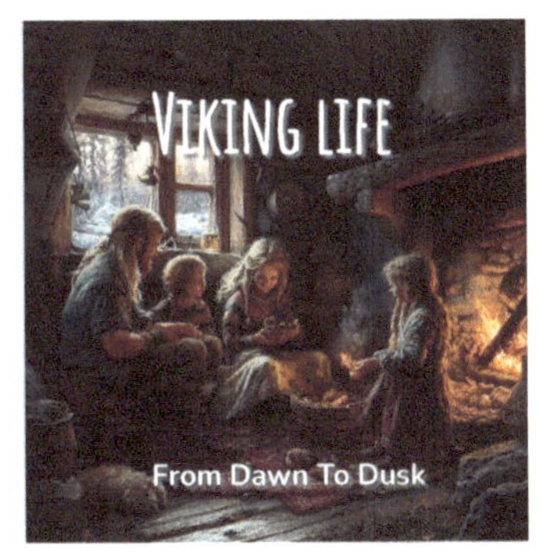

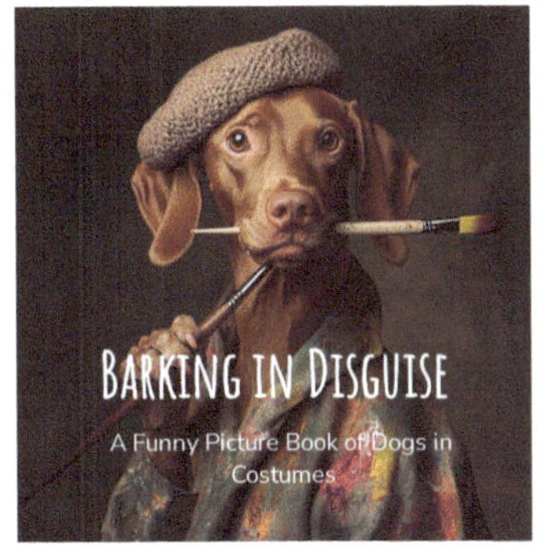

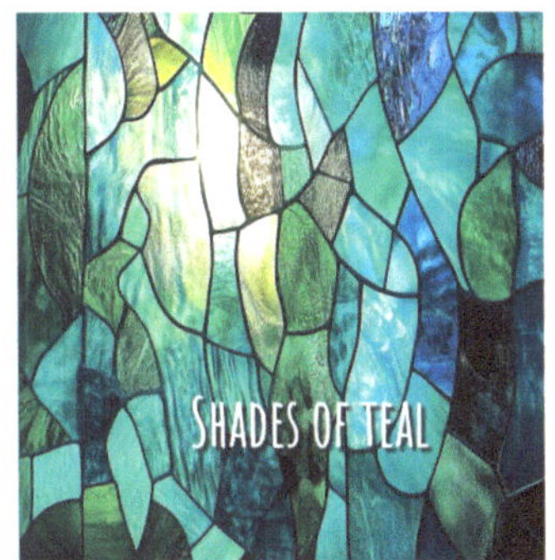

In 2020, all of a sudden, I wasn't able to go downtown anymore to do my usual street photography. After two months I was losing my mind and decided to start driving around to see if I found anything interesting to photograph through the driver side window.

I wasn't looking for anything specific; I just had this idea of photographing the area around where I live. I think you can be forgiven for thinking these photos look an awful lot like where you live. As an American I'm sure you'll recognize the strip malls, the stroads, the fast food, the power lines, the flags, and the cars.

By the time I had taken enough photos to feel like there weren't any more to take, I ended up shooting and developing 50 rolls of Fujifilm Provia positive slide film, both 35mm and 120 formats.

As I looked through all the photos I had taken in a three year time period, I kept seeing the same themes pop up, all relating to the inherent inhumanity that appears to be baked into our society. As far as I can tell it's because our society is built solely around the idea of maximizing profit for those in power and never using our resources just for the public good.

I hate that the photos which speak to me from this series are so bleak, but this is what I see. None of this is intended as art; it's intended as a record of American society at this moment from my point of view.

I encourage all those who view this book to see it as inspiration for change to a more human focused society. Remember, the most powerful things we have in America are how we vote at the ballot box and how we vote with our wallets.

Jon

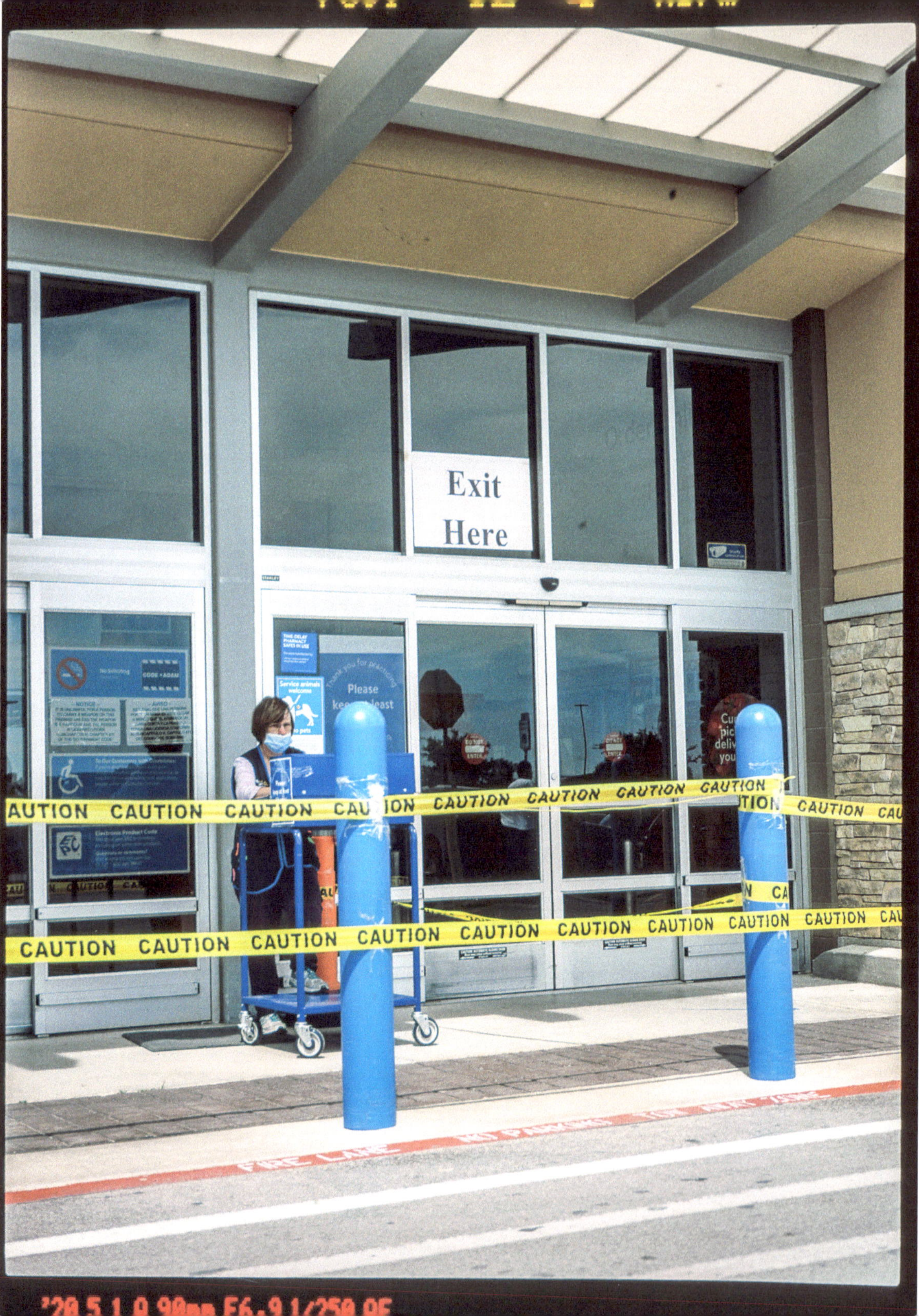

Exit
Here
CAUTION CAUTION CAUTION CAUTION CAUTION CAUTION CAUTION CAUTION CAUTION CAUTION
CAUTION CAUTION CAUTION CAUTION CAUTION CAUTION CAUTION CAUTION CAUTION
No Soliciting
Service animals welcome
Please keep pets at least

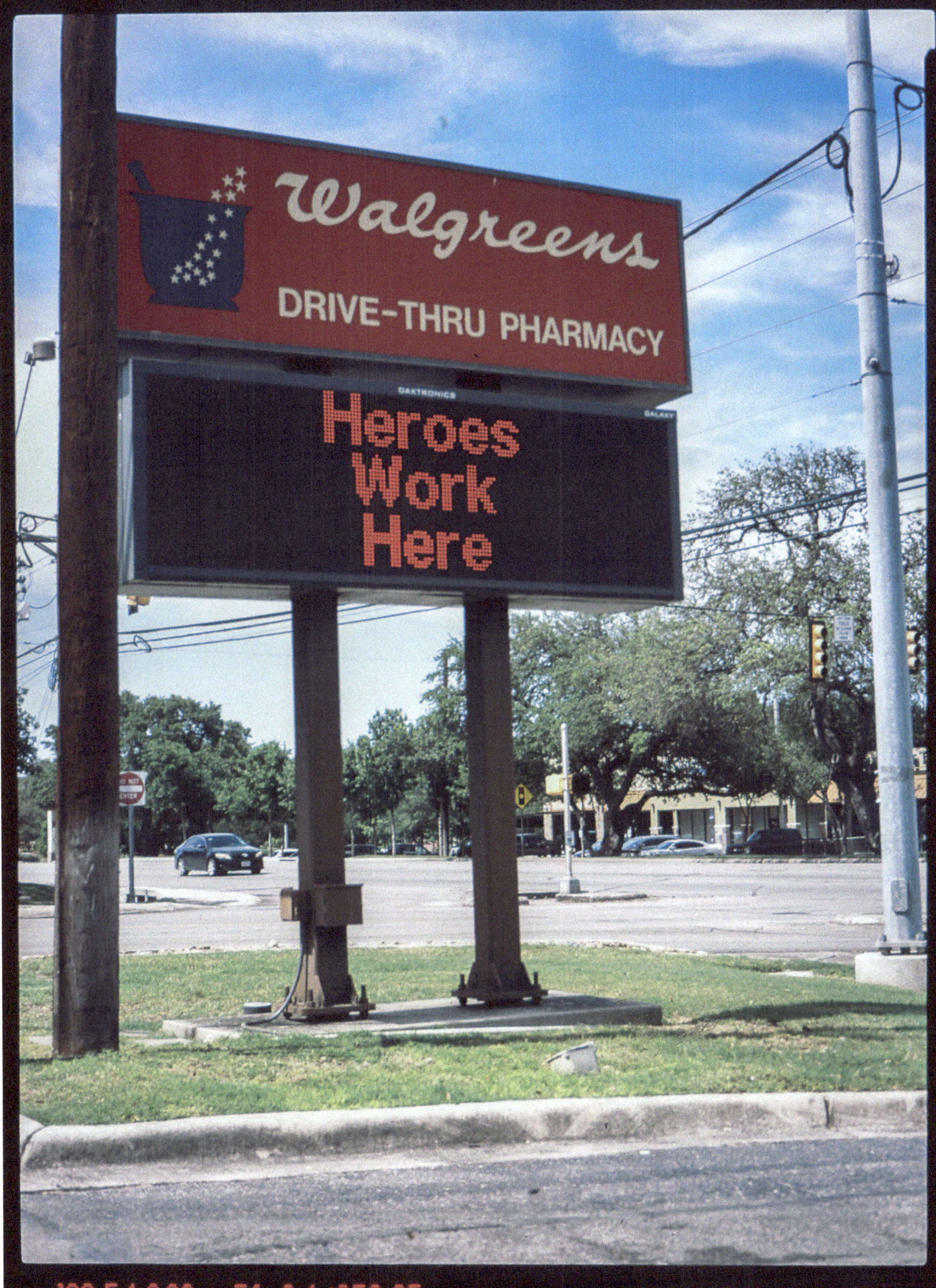

Walgreens
DRIVE-THRU PHARMACY
DAKTRONICS
GALAXY
Heroes
Work
Here

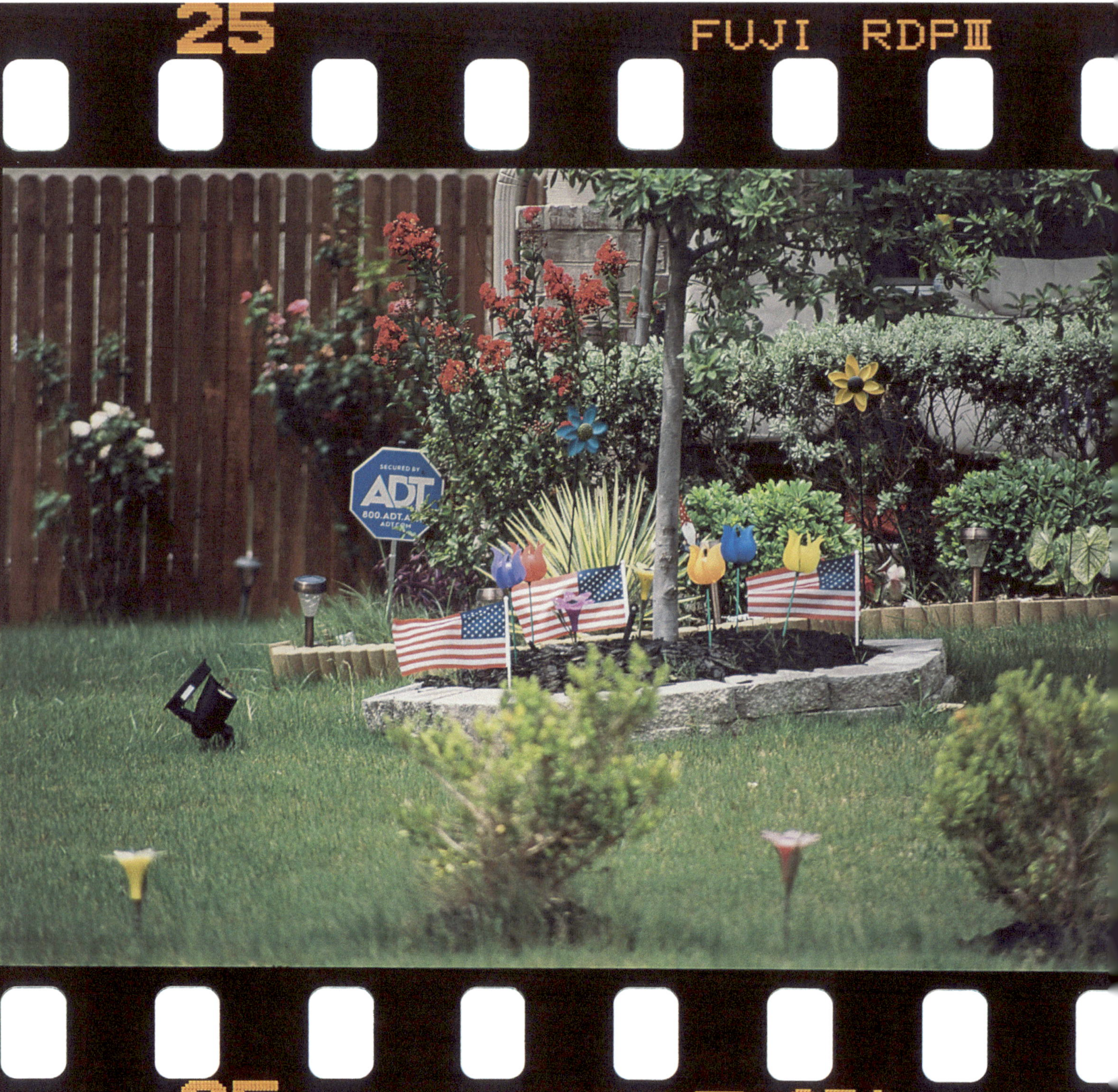
25
FUJI RDPⅢ
SECURED BY
ADT
800.ADT.A
ADT.com
25
36
25A